Humanizing Nursing Education

A Confluent Approach Through Group Process

Humanizing Nursing Education

A Confluent Approach Through Group Process

Virginia G. King, R.N., M.S.
Assistant Professor of Nursing Education,
Norwalk Community College, Norwalk, Connecticut

Norma A. Gerwig, R.N., M.A.
Assistant Professor of Nursing Education,
Norwalk Community College, Norwalk, Connecticut

Nursing Resources
An information activity of Concept Development, Inc.
Wakefield, Massachusetts

Table of Contents

Preface

Traditionally, nursing education has employed a didactic approach to teaching. Emphasis has been placed solely on the cognitive aspects of learning—structure and content—and not on the actual process. Typically, a body of significant information is presented by the teacher to the student. The student is then expected to assimilate said information and apply it appropriately. Cognitive (or informative) teaching is one-sided, inflexible and limited, in that it totally ignores the affective aspects of learning. The authors feel that this type of autocratic education is dehumanizing to the learner and has had a dehumanizing effect on the entire practice of nursing.

The goal of this book is to humanize nursing education, because total development—cognitive and affective—is essential to the nurse, in order for her effectively to respond to experiences intellectually, emotionally, and physically. Therefore, as nurse educators, we must deal with the student as a "whole person," not merely as a cognitive being. We believe this end can be accomplished through the use of a humanistic approach to nursing education.

Humanistic education goes beyond cognitive education. It is education for living. It provides a means whereby students are encouraged to develop toward living self-actualizing and responsible lives, realizing both their cognitive and affective potential.

This book demonstrates how nursing education can be humanized by using a combined learning theory consisting of a Gestalt approach, confluent education and group process. This approach evolved from the authors' decision to explore and implement a method of teaching and learning acceptable, meaningful and helpful to nursing students and to ourselves as teachers.

The first component of this combined theory, a Gestalt approach, fosters development of the principles of awareness, openness, uniqueness, and personal responsibility through an experiential mode of learning. In experiential learning, the whole person—intellectual, emotional, and development of the principles of awareness, openness, uniqueness, and personal responsibility through an experiential mode of learning. In experiential learning, the whole person—intellectual, emotional, and physical—is an integral part of the learning event. Although the stimulus may come from external sources, the learning experience is self-initiated. The sense of discovery, of reaching out, and of understanding arises from within the individual student.

The second component, confluent education, is person-centered education rather than skill- or content-centered. It involves the flowing together of mind and feelings. It is very much akin to what in "creative theory" is called the "aha" experience, the moment of insight and recognition when, after the collection of unrelated data, a pattern of recognition is suddenly seen.

The third component and also the medium for promoting experiential learning is group process. It is our premise that learning is a social process enhanced by the interpersonal relations, optimal communication skills, and group dynamics. The idea that education is critically dependent on communication and interaction between people emphasizes to us the need for a teacher to foster dynamic interplay between people through the facilitation of group process.

It is our belief that the three components of this combined learning theory will humanize nursing education by personalizing and deepening the students' experience, furthering the development of their wholeness, and helping them to fulfill their individual potential for both cognitive and affective growth.

In this educational approach, the teacher becomes a facilitator of learning rather than a disseminator of information. The roles of teacher and student become interdependent. Full expression and sharing of feelings and ideas among students is encouraged. Students are motivated to work enthusiastically and independently toward their full learning potential.

This book is written for nurse educators, especially clinical nursing instructors and graduate level nursing students, to introduce them to the confluent approach to nursing education through group process. It is the authors' hope that this book will motivate and encourage nurse educators, present and future, to incorporate this innovation into their teaching and thereby humanize nursing education. With slight modifications, this approach could also be used in the areas of continuing education, patient education, and nursing management.

Our experience with combined learning theory has been stimulating and exciting for teacher and student alike. The students exhibited a new interest and responsibility toward their learning. By sharing their individual concepts, feelings, and ideas with their peers, they were able to broaden their own concepts, heighten their feelings of self-worth as contributing members, and develop their communication skills.

As teachers, we have found this new and dynamic learning process allows us unlimited originality and scope to develop our teaching potential to the fullest. We are challenged, enthusiastic, and most eager to share our feelings, experiences, and conclusions with you, the reader.

Objectives

The reader will:

1. Gain information about the humanistic philosophy of education.

2. Become aware of the need for and value of a humanistic approach to nursing education.

3. Become knowledgeable about confluent education.

4. Define the role of the facilitator in managing group process.

5. Define the role of the student in group process.

6. Gain knowledge of the implementation of confluent education through group process in nursing education.

7. Share the experience of group process as presented in situations describing actual applications of confluent education.

8. Be able to recognize impediments to the accomplishment of group goals.

9. Be able to implement a variety of techniques to foster a confluent approach to learning.

10. Be motivated and encouraged to try a confluent approach to nursing education through group process.

Acknowledgments

We would like to acknowledge and express our sincere thanks to Mrs. Norma Albrecht, our typist, grammar and spelling expert and generally an invaluable individual with regard to the completion of our manu-script. She spent many, many hours working on our behalf, and we are deeply grateful.

We would also like to thank our families who, in spite of many prolonged phone calls, innumerable "pot luck" dinners, and oftentimes a general preoccupation on our parts, were always supportive and understanding, and ever ready to offer an encouraging word when one was sorely needed.

We would also like to acknowledge the professional assistance afforded us by the staff of the Norwalk Community College Library, the Fairfield University Library, the Norwalk Board of Education Professional Library, and the Greenwich Public Library.

CHAPTER 1

A Humanistic Philosophy of Education

In this chapter we would like to familiarize you with our philosophy concerning the nature of people, their growth, and how they make decisions about themselves, because this philosophy forms the foundation on which we have developed our approach to teaching. This philosophy brought about the change in our teaching style, from being didactic, directive teachers controlling the learners, to continually striving to facilitate the process of learning. Our philosophy is basically a humanistic one. This is of particular importance to us, because it means that a major goal of our teaching is to enhance a student's individual potential and responsibility for personal growth.

Because our philosophy is derived from humanistic psychology, we are providing a background in this discipline. We will explore its development and its contributions to the study of humans and their adaptation to the environment. In later chapters we will show how education uses these principles to enhance the process of man's adaptation to his environment.

OVERVIEW OF HUMANISTIC PSYCHOLOGY

Prior to the introduction of humanism, psychology was dominated by two major theories of human behavior: psychoanalysis (Freudianism) and behaviorism. Humanistic psychology has grown in large measure in reaction to the seeming inadequacy of these theories to deal with the higher nature, or humanness, of people[23]. Freudianism has dealt for the most part with unconscious behavior and pathological personality development, while behaviorism has centered on research related to the environment and its control of human behavior through conditioning.

Humanistic psychology differs vastly from both. It not only promotes an eclectic, integrative interpretation of human growth and development, which supplements and builds on these other theories, it also offers feasible alternatives to some of the approaches to understanding humans that have been generated by

1

them. As demonstrated in Maslow's hierarchy of human needs [5, p. 50], humanistic psychology emphasizes healthy personality development instead of pathological personality development. It concentrates on conscious rather than on unconscious behavior. Furthermore, opposing the theory of environmental control, humanistic psychology features elements of Maslow's theory of motivation [9], Rogers' theory of self-determinism [3] and Glasser's theory of individual responsibility [4].

It also emphasizes a phenomenological approach to the study of human consciousness. This scientific method describes and classifies, but does not interpret, phenomena such as human experience as it is known through the senses. Research investigations have led to identification of elements in human relations that foster growth and development, thereby expanding the strictly objective methodology used by behaviorists to study human behavior[16, pp. 98–103; 18].

Major Differences Between Humanistic Psychology and Psychoanalytic Theory

The field of psychology has come a long distance since the development of psychoanalysis. It is helpful to have an understanding of the concepts of psychoanalysis and the major ways in which it differs from humanistic psychology in order to understand the full scope of the latter and its implications for all of society, especially education.

Sigmund Freud is responsible for the development of psychoanalytic theory, one of history's most comprehensive and influential theories of human behavior. It has been pervasive and has dominated not only the field of psychotherapy, but most other areas of our culture, including education and child-rearing. Psychoanalytic theory has helped make people aware of the value of studying child development[6].

Freud's interest centered on people who were mentally disturbed. These patients comprised his laboratory subjects for study and research. Through the study of their pathological behavior, he formed theories to explain that behavior's origins. Freud stressed the influence of the unconscious mind on human behavior and personality development. To him, the unconscious mind is made up of the id, ego and superego. These elements must be in reasonable balance to maintain psychological health and acceptable personality adjustment.

The id represents life's instincts for survival and propagation. Id instincts are described as being aggressive, powerful, antisocial and irrational. They are the motivation behind human behavior. Laws of reason or logic do not govern the id. The id does not possess values, ethics or morality, but is motivated by one force only: to obtain immediate satisfaction of the instinctual needs of an organism. Its goal is to release tension through reflex activity or wish fulfillment [6, pp. 22–26]. An individual's id is believed to be in constant conflict with the superego, which represents the social conscience, or moral code, and the social responsibility imposed by parents and society. The superego is the internalizing of the ideal rather than the real. An overdeveloped or an underdeveloped super-ego can lead to problems in personality development.

The ego determines actions or behavior by controlling or balancing the forces of conflict between the id and superego. Ego activity is governed by the reality principle, the purpose of which is to postpone the discharge of energy or release of tension until an appropriate object on which to do so is available. To be appropriate, an object must both satisfy a specific need and be socially acceptable [6, p. 28]. According to Freudian theory, a person can become mentally ill when the conflict between an overdeveloped or unrealistic superego and the powerful instinctual drives of the id remain unresolved and become overwhelming. Ultimately, there is inability to cope with the resulting stress[5]. The person needs outside assistance in dealing with the illness.

Two of the tools developed by psychoanalytic theory for treating mental illness are free association and dream analysis. Through these techniques, Freud encouraged individuals to recall and explore their childhood memories. While he listened to their recollections and interpreted their dreams, he was able to achieve insight into the development of their personalities. Eventually, through this process guilt feelings were reduced and the patient would develop the ability to sublimate or channel repressed desires of the id into socially acceptable outlets. This resolved the overwhelming conflict between his id and superego. The patient thereby conquered and eliminated the mental disturbance[6].

Maslow went beyond psychoanalytic theory to form a broader, more comprehensive theory of healthy human development. Within this concept, Freudian psychotherapy was identified as an important means of communication, and basic biological needs became the foundation of a hierarchy of needs leading to self-actualization that are positive motivative forces for growth.

Maslow[9] differed greatly from Freud because he believed that, in order to understand mental illness or pathological human growth and development, one must first understand healthy growth and development. He felt that concentrated study of the insane, the neurotic, the psychopath, the criminal, the delinquent and the feeble-minded could not help but influence the development of a stunted, limited, one-sided psychology and philosophy. Maslow studied the best human beings he could find. This orientation provided quite different aspects of human behavior for observation than those examined by Freud. From his study, Maslow developed a hierarchy of basic human needs, which includes environmental, physiological and growth needs. This hierarchy of needs formed the framework for a holistic approach to the study of a person's growth toward self-actualization. Maslow's hierarchy helps us to realize that Freud's level of basic physical needs and the level of self-actualization do not contradict each other. Fulfillment of one level of need is a necessary step before moving on to the next level. When the first level is gratified it disappears and evolves to the next level. As for motivation, the achievement of one need does not bring about a state of rest, but rather a desire to fulfill the need at the next higher level[9, pp. 26-31].

In harmony with Maslow's growth potential philosophy, Rogers[3, p. lxxiv] suggests, "We might then value: man as a process of becoming, as a process of achieving worth and dignity through the development of his potentialities; the individual human being as a self-actualizing process, moving on to more challenging and enriching experiences; the process by which the individual creatively adapts to an ever-new and changing world; the process by which knowledge transcends itself . . .." As an alternative to mental illness as it is construed in psychoanalytic theory, Rogers[3] presents the humanistic concept that ideally the organism is always endeavoring to actualize itself. A problem occurs when the self becomes static. The person then experiences maladjustment. Even if this happens, Rogers indicates that only the individual knows what hurts, what directions to go in, what problems are crucial, what experiences are deeply buried [3, p. xxix] and thus people can and should be trusted to direct their own lives [3, p. xli]. Rogers supports Maslow's concept of motivation, saying that every organism has a tendency to maintain, to enhance and to reproduce itself[3, p. 5].

In his concepts of reality therapy, Glasser[4] departs even further from traditional psychoanalytic theory. He and others believe that mental illness is caused by an inability on the part of the individual to fulfill the essential basic needs for relatedness and respect at the interpersonal, social level of functioning. This theory differs radically from the Freudian view that mental illness is caused by an inability of the person to meet, in a socially acceptable way, basic physical (id) needs of sex and aggression because of an overdeveloped or underveloped superego. Glasser[4] theorizes that, in order for an individual to fulfill his inherent needs of relatedness and respect, he must learn to do what is realistic, responsible and right. It is when a person does not or cannot learn that problems occur. Individual responsibility for need fulfillment is a central concept in reality therapy. It is defined as the ability to fulfill one's needs and to do so in a way that will not interfere with another person's ability to do the same. A person who lacks responsibility is unable to fulfill the needs for loving and being loved, for having feelings of self-worth and the feeling of being worthwhile to others. If this happens, the person will eventually become ill or suffer or cause others to suffer. In other words, irresponsible behavior in people causes illness. People do not behave irresponsibly because they are ill. Glasser believes there is no such thing as mental illness (as defined by Freud), only irresponsibility or irresponsible behavior.

On this foundation, Glasser[4] elaborates on six major areas of significant differences between what is accepted as conventional Freudian-based psychoanalytic therapy and reality therapy. The points are summarized as follows:

1. Conventional psychiatry believes in the concept of mental illness. It attempts to classify people according to type of illness and to treat them appropriately. Reality therapy does not recognize mental illness. Therefore an individ-

ual cannot become involved in therapy as a mentally ill patient, and by so doing, avoid responsibility for his behavior.

2. A vital part of conventional psychiatric treatment is probing into a patient's past history, searching for insights into an understanding of the cause of the patient's problem. Reality therapy accepts that the past cannot be changed; it works with people in the present. Learning responsible behavior is what is critical, not recording past events and irresponsible behavior. It also does not accept that people are limited by the past. It rejects traditional psychoanalytic approaches to psychotherapy.

3. Transference plays a central role in conventional psychiatry. The patient is supposed to transfer the feelings and attitudes once held for significant people in the past to the therapist. The therapist then relives with the patient those past problems, indicating when the patient is repeating the same inadequate behavior with the therapist. This interaction helps the patient to gain insight into old attitudes and feelings and to learn to relate to people in a more effective way. Reality therapists relate to people as themselves, in the present, not as transference figures.

4. Conventional psychotherapy emphasizes that insight into the unconscious mind is essential for therapy to be successful. Reality therapy does not look for unconscious conflicts or the reasons for them, because it does not excuse a patient's behavior on the basis of unconscious motivation.

5. Deviant behavior is considered by conventional psychiatry to be a product of mental illness. When mental illness is cured the behavior will then be in accordance with the rules of society. Until then, a patient is not held responsible for his behavior. Reality therapists emphasize the morality of behavior, the need to face the issues of right and wrong, feeling it enhances the involvement of the patient with the therapist. Reality therapists believe that irresponsible behavior by the patient has caused the problems.

6. Conventional psychiatry does not teach patients. It assumes that once patients understand both the historical and unconscious sources of their problems that they will learn better behavior. Reality therapy teaches patients better, more responsible ways to fulfill their needs. This can only be done when there is proper and sufficient involvement in the relationship between the therapist and the patient, so that the patient experiences that a person whom he genuinely cares about, genuinely cares about him.

This brief presentation has highlighted and summarized some of the major differences between the views of human behavior that are manifested by Freudian theory and those found in present-day humanistic psychology. The application of these humanistic views to education, especially to our concept of nursing education, will be elaborated on later.

Major Differences Between Humanistic Psychology and Behaviorism

The core issue separating humanistic psychology from behaviorism is the question of who or what controls human behavior. Are we proactive or reactive to our environment? How this issue is resolved influences one's ultimate philosophy of human potential. Eventually, this resolution affects education and the way we approach the learning process.

Watson is recognized as the founder of behaviorism because he developed its basic concepts and initiated the use of the word *behaviorism.* His work was originally influenced by Pavlov's model of classical conditioning, which he accepted as the basic rationale for learning. He built on this model, however, and became the promoter of the concepts of conditioned reflex and environmentalism. He fostered the idea that individual differences are caused by experiences rather than genetics[7]. In the context of environmentalism, learning may be defined as a consistent change in behavior that results from an organism's interaction with the environment. The behavioral changes may be observed in the realms of cognitive, affective or psychomotor development.

While B. F. Skinner accepted the theories of classical stimulus/response conditioning[7, pp. 46–47], he extended them further with the development of a theory known as operant conditioning. Consider as an example, a rat in a cage who, when running around, presses a lever. For his unsolicited lever-pressing action, he receives a food pellet, which serves as a reward and increases the probability that he will repeat the action. In operant conditioning, behaviors (such as the rat's lever-pressing) that arise from within an organism and are not solicited by any known stimuli are called "operants," because they are operations or actions performed on the environment by an organism. The reward (the food pellet) that an organism receives from the environment as a result of operant behavior serves as a stimulus for this behavior to occur again. This is called "operant conditioning" as opposed to Watson's "respondant conditioning," in which the organism is reacting to a known stimulus from the environment. In either case, reinforcement or lack of reinforcement has a great deal to do with controlling the kind of behavior in which an individual engages. In fact, it is Skinner's contention[22] that humans are clearly controlled by the environment through the effects of both kinds of conditioning, which make us reactive to that environment.

Humanistic psychology refutes the idea of absolute environmental control over human behavior. Although it recognizes that there are external forces that motivate behavior and that a person is affected by environment, the concept of environmental control is integrated into an expanded view of humans. This view emphasizes the theory that motivation for growth toward becoming self-actualized is inherent in an organism. We are considered always to be striving to reach this level. The various processes that bring us toward this ultimate level of self-actualization are defined as growth[9]. These growth processes occur continually throughout life, not only to accomplish the progressive fulfillment of basic physical and emotional needs to the point where they no longer exist, but also to fulfill needs beyond these in the realms of talent and other creative capacities and potentials.

A second aspect of the humanistic expanded view of man encompasses Rogers' theory of self-determinism, in which he states that a person can understand those factors from the past that have contributed to who he is and can move on to choose his own future [3, p. 75]. This theory clearly says that an individual can go beyond merely responding to and being controlled by the environment.

Glasser [4] stresses that people are basically responsible for themselves and their behavior, and for evaluating it. He says that a person is not controlled by environment, is not merely reactive to it. Each of us has the ability to evaluate our own behavior and, having evaluated it, can make decisions about it and take action to improve it where it is below standards. The more responsible we are in doing this, the more control we have over ourselves and our destiny.

The implication derived from studying who or what controls human behavior is that education must not only abide by the principles of learning theory arising from behaviorism, but transcend them by adding a humanistic dimension that will help the individual grow to be a more fully functioning, self-actualizing and responsible person, able to direct his life effectively and independently.

Aim of Humanistic Psychology

The aim of this branch of psychology is to promote the full development of human potential. Because it is person-centered, it places the utmost value on the dignity of the human being. It stresses self-realization and self-actualization as the goals of human development. As we have seen, it offers as models the "fully functioning" [15], "self-actualized" [9] or "responsible" [4] person.

The characteristics of this kind of person are well described by Maslow [5]. Everything that you can imagine that is good or right about a person seems to apply to people who are self-actualizing, fully functioning and responsible. They are mature, competent and stable. They are humble and able to listen carefully to other people, admitting that they do not know everything, that they are always learning. These individuals are involved and committed to work that is done well and to the best of their ability; they are open to change and are not threatened by it as rigid inflexible people are.

These people are inner directed and less needful of honors, prestige and rewards. They have an inner sense of psychological freedom. They have the strength to be contrary to their culture and society when they believe basic principles are being violated. Their value systems are stable. They feel a kinship with all human beings and a responsibility for and commitment beyond fulfilling their own needs to solving the problems of society. These people accept themselves and their natures. They are able to enjoy other people, accepting them as they are, recognizing in them their own separate individual potential for growth. They develop and maintain harmonious relationships with other people that are non-exploitive, but are instead deep, respectful and loving, and facilitate each other's growth potential.

What Has Humanistic Psychology Done?

Humanistic psychology has not only developed a positive growth-oriented dimension of psychology, it has established what is essential for enhancing this optimal growth process so that an individual can be assisted in growing toward becoming a fully functioning, responsible and self-actualizing person[2, pp. 358–392; 24, pp. 80–143]. Phenomenological research studies of therapeutic relationships have established that a primary agent for influencing change and personal growth is the degree to which that individual experiences certain qualities such as warmth, empathy and congruence in his relationship with the person who is trying to help him[16, pp. 98–103; 18]. The presence of these qualities within a therapeutic relationship provides the kind of non-threatening climate that will enable a person to get in touch with himself and with his inherent drive toward self-actualization.

Humanistic psychology realizes that self-actualization does not take place in a protected, isolated vacuum, but that societal conditions play a significant role in influencing human growth and development. This awareness has motivated humanistic psychologists to take the principles learned from studying therapeutic relationships that facilitate growth, and apply them toward social institutions. Humanizing institutions has become a way to accomplish the ultimate aim of humanistic psychology, which is the fullest possible development of human potential.

The application of these principles to the process of learning has led to the development of a humanistic approach to education.

HUMANISTIC EDUCATION

Definition and Concepts

Humanistic education is education of the total person. It allows the learner to realize and develop his full potentialities, going beyond basic cognitive learning into the realm of affective learning: What do I think? What do I feel? What is the significance of this learning experience to me? How does it help me grow as a person?

If you accept the premise that the learner is always in a state of becoming and that we are all learners throughout our entire lives, the scope of humanistic education is infinite. In comparison, the scope of traditional, didactic, teacher-oriented education is limited. Its major concern is to impart cognitive knowledge to create the so-called educated person, but this ignores the entire affective realm of humans.

Humanistic education is person-centered. The person is helped to recognize and develop his own unique potentialities, facilitating the process of individual growth and positive behavioral changes through active learner participation. The student goes beyond merely responding to environment, to identifying a role within it and determining ways to influence or change it. As a consequence of direct involvement in the learning process, recognition of self-worth, personal needs and means of self-fulfillment become apparent. William Glasser[4] says that a person has the potential for learning to be responsible for fulfilling his personal needs of loving and being loved, for feeling worthwhile to himself and to others, and for doing this without interfering with other people's abilities to fulfill their own needs. He also stresses that people have the ability for both self-evaluation and self-control and must exercise these abilities in order to fulfill the need to be worthwhile[4, p. 10]. Meaningful learning is a matter of self-responsibility and is basically self-directed. The learner must define his own learning needs and be assisted to find a personalized way in which to meet them. The teacher becomes the person who helps him find the way, and therefore facilitates the learning process; but the learner personalizes it.

This type of approach integrates all learning (cognitive, affective and psycho-motor) in a manner meaningful to the learner, in order to foster efficient personalization of the content with subsequent behavioral changes that enhance and improve the learner's total being.

Learning that is self-directed is individualized and significant. If the learner is allowed the freedom of personal choice in the educative process and is allowed to answer the voice from within that says, "What are my needs and how can I meet them in a way that helps me cope with today, prepare better for tomorrow and become a balanced responsible person?," he will be afforded the opportunity to grow toward becoming a total, self-actualizing person. Throughout this growth process, the affective/emotional skills and abilities will be developed, as will the cognitive and psychomotor ones. In true learning, all of the senses are involved and contribute to the learning process.

What makes humanistic education different is that the individual's purposes and goals come from within, the learning experience is self-initiated and the learner is responsible for his own learning. Rogers[17, p. 487] says, "The organism has one basic tendency and striving . . . to actualize, maintain, and enhance the experiencing organism." If we accept this premise of a basic human striving, our educative efforts must be directed toward providing means for maintenance and enhancement of the individual student. The educative process then hinges on what the individual student perceives as significant to his preservation and to his striving for completeness or self-actualization.

Problems with Traditional Education

Traditional education has historically set teaching goals and instituted a wide variety of teaching methods in order to attain them. The didactic teacher strives toward a teacher-defined goal, molding and reshaping students into preconceived specifications and standards. The end product, the so-called educated person, is a figment of the teacher's perception, a teacher-defined product. The humanity in such a system is absent. Too often the teacher's perceptions, needs and goals dominate the classroom, obscuring the student's motivations to the point that the student finally surrenders. He is forced to learn according to the teacher's perception of what is significant to know and how to use what is being taught. If the material being taught is not seen as relevant by the student, meaningful learning does not take place. The student cannot be expected just to accept the material being taught; he must be allowed to view the material through his own perception, to determine its relevance and how it will enhance his being.

Silberman observes, "Most teachers dominate the classroom, giving students no option except that of passivity"[20,pp. 148-149].The teacher initiates or controls two-thirds to three-quarters of all classroom communication. When the student speaks he usually is responding to a teacher-initiated question[20, p. 149]. The I-Thou relationship is at a minimum in the traditional classroom. The student is not recognized as a unique human being, but as a controlled thing; I speak and you listen, I ask a question and you provide an answer, preferably the right one. The teacher makes certain statements, the student records them, regurgitates them at the proper testing time and forgets them. He is not allowed to internalize, question, fit the facts into his perception of the greater whole and thereby accept, reject or modify their impact with regard to his own needs and goals.

How often have you attended an opening day class when the teacher says, "You will be responsible for your own learning. You will only get out of this course what you put into it." The teacher then proceeds totally to dominate the remaining semester with endless lectures, preselected films and "significant" assignments. The assumption is that only the teacher knows what the student needs to know to "make it" in life. The original statement the teacher made is borne out. The student gets little or nothing out of the course because he is not allowed any original input. He is not allowed his individuality, his freedom to learn. Everything is presented from the teacher's perception to meet the teacher's teaching needs. The student is left out.

It hardly seems possible that education was intended to be imparted in this manner. There are a great number of dedicated, sincere teachers in our school systems, colleges and universities who would be appalled at the description of the traditional classroom just presented, but when there is genuine examination of the amount of actual educational freedom, most would have to agree it is limited. Time, standardization of curriculum, and teacher/student ratios are usually the reasons given for this lack. The teacher does not have time for each and every student and so must teach to a nonexistent "average" student level. If the teacher would employ a humanistic form of teaching, in other words, *stop* teaching and start facilitating learning, the problem of individualized education would take care of itself.

A major criticism of learning institutions today is that they are dehumanized, and that the educative process is dehumanizing to students and teachers alike. Benne suggests several major barriers to humanized education that are relevant to a proposal for its implementation. Let us consider two of these. First he states, "Schooling is seen and practiced as a process in which the 'correct' environmental influences, predetermined by adults, are brought to bear upon assumedly passive and plastic learners to produce the educational 'products' needed by 'society' "[1, p. 47].

Second, he speaks of "the idolatry of intellectualism" wherein "the thinking of men and women is separated radically from the living contexts, internal and external, of the human organism. Intellect is separated from feeling, emotion, and volition"[1, p. 47].

While both these areas have already been discussed, it is worth taking a second look at two major factors in today's educational system that dramatically point out the need to humanize it. One is that most decisions regarding the student's educational needs are made by supposedly enlightened educators with virtually no input from the student recipient. The student is something that is fed the information necessary to convert him into an acceptable product. The other is that the necessary information received is totally cognitive. How does one function as a total person in society when only one's intellect has been educated? One can only assume from Benne's description that the plastic learner of today becomes the plastic society member of tomorrow, dehumanized, with no spontaneous expression of feelings, attitudes, values and perceptions, but simply a shiny surface reflecting the environment.

Humanizing Education

How can we as educators help humanize education? What alternatives are available? Rogers states, "The goal of education in general must be to develop a society in which people can live more comfortably with change than with rigidity"[15, p. 304]. This raises a problem with traditional education. How can an ability to adapt to and live with change be learned in a rigid inflexible classroom environment? The very concept of change implies creativity, original thought, sharing and synthesizing ideas and feelings, values and perceptions. The classroom is bursting with unique contributions; we need to foster the sharing of these and avoid having all eyes and ears focused on the figure at the front of the room. Teacher-centered education allows for only one-directional communication.

To alter this, Rogers[15, p. 304] says that a way must be found to develop a climate in the classroom in which the focus is not on the teacher and teaching, but on the facilitation of significant self-directed learning initiated by the student. He also contends that the facilitation of significant learning depends on certain qualities of attitude that exist in the personal relationship between the facilitator and the learner[8, p. 65].

Benne offers a humanistic alternative of a "community" sense of learning. "Community, in a normative sense of that term, is an association of people mutually and reciprocally involved with each other, caring for each other, aware of the human effects of their decisions and actions upon those within and outside the association, and committed to being responsible for these effects"[1, p. 55]. This statement aptly describes humanistic education: a community or group involvement of teachers and students, with all members sharing a sense of responsibility for their own individual learning and for the learning of the group, all members giving and taking, interacting with their contributions to help clarify and increase understanding among all members of the group. Thus while each member of the group contributes to the whole, he retains his individuality and fosters his individual growth through worthwhile involvement in activities that add to his understanding, afford him expression of his feelings in his own way and help him develop self-awareness and clarify his values as he moves toward self-actualization.

We must look at the goals of humanistic education. Its specific major goal is to create the self-actualized person. This goal is actually unattainable, for in reality humanistic education at best creates a person constantly striving toward becoming self-actualized. But the person who moves in this direction is humane, open and receptive to change. He thinks, feels and acts not only on the basis of intellect, but also on feelings. He understands, respects and accepts others and himself. He is a responsible person, fully functioning, spontaneous and creative, always involved in the process of self-education[12, pp. 21–22].

If humanistic education is to help the student move toward self-actualization, behavioral changes must occur during and as a result of education. Behavioral changes on the learner's part occur when education is relevant and meaningful to him. Thus in order to change behavior we must first change perceptions. If the learner sees positive indications for himself in the learning experience, and the experience is inconsistent with but non-threatening to his self-concept, behavioral changes will occur; learning will take place[12, p. 69].

Valett [25, pp. 53–54] suggests a different humanistic approach using a five-level affective educational program with a major affective behavioral goal at each level, from which specific objectives or learning activities may be developed to help the learner accomplish the goal. These goals are as follows:

Level 1: Understanding basic human needs
Level 2: Expressing human feelings
Level 3: Self-awareness and control

Level 4: Becoming aware of human values
Level 5: Developing social and personal maturity

A program based on these goals would be meaningful to the learner, allow for individual expression, help him develop self-awareness, identify his basic and inherent needs and cope with his feelings; however, this approach deals with the student's affective needs only, and does not afford a learning experience that creates the total person. The teaching method that is discussed in this book incorporates these goals as an integral part of cognitive-affective learning as it relates to nursing education.

The success of a humanistic educational experience rests heavily on the climate of the learning environment, that is, the relationship of the teacher and the student. The whole tone of such an experience begins with the teacher[10]. The teacher's attitude and behavior serve as the role model of a self-actualized person. Tageson says, "We 'teach' respect for self and others by respecting self and others, by creating an atmosphere in which such values are constantly lived out, displayed in all our relationships, and experienced consistently by all concerned" [23, p. 95]. Thus the task to humanize education begins with the teacher. For the traditional didactic teacher this may seem like an overwhelming change. Becoming a more humanistic teacher can be frightening as well as challenging, but also rewarding. Yet the basic conditions necessary to create and maintain the type of personal relationship identified in humanistic education are inherent in many motivated, flexible teachers. These are: empathy, respect (warmth) and genuineness. Patterson feels that these three basic attributes are necessary to establish conditions that "minimize threat in interpersonal relationships, and . . . lead to the positive changes in behavior which are characteristics of self-actualizing persons"[12, p. 70].

Empathy in humanistic education means that the teacher has an understanding of things from the student's frame of reference. The teacher is able to view the situation as if he were the student. Empathic understanding might simply be defined as understanding derived as one wears another's shoes. True empathic understanding, however, is not simple and is an enviable personality trait that must be purposefully developed. One can relate to the empathic person with ease because "he understands and cares."

The second trait, respect, means the teacher accepts students as they are, without judgment, and likes them as people. This is the teacher who wants to see his students reach their own self-determined goals and find fulfillment.

The teacher who is genuine is sincere, says what he thinks and means it. There is no artificiality about him. Genuineness implies honesty and trustworthiness.

Thus the teacher must possess and model empathy toward students, respect students and be genuine in order to establish a helping relationship with them that will assist them with their growth[14]. This will create a learning climate that will foster the development of these same traits in the students. "The conditions and the goal are the same"[12, p. 73].

The conditions that allow for freedom of learning, individuality of expression and personal growth do so because the teacher-student relationship and the learning environment are non-threatening. At the same time, they foster the development of these attributes within the student. They work because the student is more relaxed, less defensive and usually feels better about himself. He is not judged. He is free objectively to assess his self-worth and pursue the development of areas in which he finds himself lacking. When the climate is relaxed, people feel free to respond and be themselves. In this atmosphere, the student can begin to realize his full potential and move toward becoming more fully functioning, self-actualizing and responsive. He will be able to respond to others on a different level, recognizing their potential for growth and helping them to grow.

REFERENCES

1. Benne, K. Humanization of schooling. *Journal of Education* 157:44–60, May 1975.
2. Berenson, B., and Carkhuff, R. *Sources of Gain in Counseling and Psychotherapy.* New York: Holt, Rinehart and Winston, 1967.
3. Evans, R. I. *Carl Rogers: The Man and His Ideas.* New York: Dutton, 1975.
4. Glasser, W. *Reality Therapy.* New York: Harper and Row, 1965.
5. Goble, F. *The Third Force.* New York: Grossman, 1970.
6. Hall, C. S. *A Primer of Freudian Psychology.* New York and Toronto: Mentor, 1954.
7. Lefrancois, G. R. *Psychology for Teaching* (2nd ed.). Belmont, Calif.: Wadsworth, 1975.
8. Lyon, H. C. *Learning to Feel—Feeling to Learn.* Columbus, Ohio: Charles E. Merrill, 1971.
9. Maslow, A. H. *Toward a Psychology of Being* (2nd ed.). New York: Van Nostrand, 1968.
10. Murray, E. Students perceptions of self-actualizaing and non self-actualizing teachers. *Journal of Teacher Education* 23:383–387, 1972.
11. Nash, P. (Ed.). Humanistic Education. *Journal of education* 157(2):1–58, 1975.
12. Patterson, C. H. *Humanistic Education.* Englewood Cliffs, N.J.: Prentice-Hall, 1973.
13. Read, D., and Simon, S. *Humanistic Education Source Book.* Englewood Cliffs, N.J.: Prentice-Hall, 1975.
14. Ripple, R. F. Affective factors influence classroom learning. *Educational Leadership* 22:476–480, 1965.
15. Rogers, C. *Client-centered Therapy: Its Current Practice, Implications and Theory.* Boston: Houghton Mifflin, 1951.
16. Rogers, C. *Freedom to Learn.* Columbus, Ohio: Charles E. Merrill, 1969.
17. Rogers, C., and Stevens, B. *Person to Person: The Problem of Being Human. A New Trend in Psychology.* Lafayette, Calif.: Real People Press, 1967.
18. Rogers, C. R. The interpersonal relationship: The core of guidance. *Harvard Educational Review* 30(4):416–429, 1962.
19. *Schools For the 70's and Beyond: A Call to Action.* Washington, D.C.: National Education Association, 1971.
20. Silberman, C. *Crisis in the Classroom.* New York: Random House, 1970.
21. Simpson, E. L., and Gray, M. *Humanistic Education: An Interpretation.* Cambridge, Mass.: Ballinger, 1976.
22. Skinner, B. F. *Walden Two* New York: Macmillan, 1948.
23. Tageson, C. W. Humanistic education. *Counseling and Values* 17(2):90–95, 1973.
24. Trauax, C. B., and Carkhuff, R. *Toward Effective Counseling and Psychotherapy.* Chicago: Aldine, 1967.
25. Valett, R. E. *Humanistic Education, Developing the Total Person.* St. Louis: Mosby, 1977.

CHAPTER 2

Humanistic Nursing Education

In this chapter we would like to review the ways in which the nurse and her role have been and are now being defined. It is our belief that today's nurse must be humanistic. Based on this belief, we feel that nursing education must teach in a humanistic manner, stressing affective as well as cognitive and psychomotor skills.

We will present a history of trends in nursing education and define what we feel is a definite need for humanism in the process.

NURSING DEFINED

One need only scan through a nursing history text to find dozens of definitions of what nursing is, how it is carried out and what its limitations are. Nurses, nurse educators, doctors and others have been defining and redefining the profession for many years.

Florence Nightingale, in 1860, believed that time, nature and the natural reparative processes of the human body rendered cure or wellness to the sick person, with minimal intervention of medical or surgical skill. In this light she felt, "What nursing has to do . . . is to put the patient in the best condition for nature to act upon him" [29, p. 133] . Miss Nightingale's broad definition of nursing still serves well.

As professionals nurses have moved away from the role of "doctors' handmaidens," and are in the process of moving through *procedure-oriented* nursing, toward *patient-centered* nursing and the emerging field of primary nursing, specialization and independent practice.

While nursing has been changing internally, everything external to it has been changing as well. Technology has advanced at a frantic pace, demanding societal and individual adjustment. Future shock is fast becoming a reality. Stress has become the major contributing factor in illness, and the ability to adapt to change is necessary for survival. The nurse today has more scientific background, more lifesaving, life-sustaining and life-recording equipment and more technology at her fingertips than ever before. She has more cognitive knowledge for dealing with the physical, mental and emotional stress of her patients. She can operate the most sophisticated computerized equipment modern health technology can provide. She is adapting and changing, keeping up with society. As nurses "we've come a long way"—or have we?

For a moment let us take a look at just how far the nurse has come since Miss Nightingale defined her role. As nursing evolved through the nineteenth and into the twentieth century, it was looked upon as an art of doing and caring. In 1934, Effie Taylor said, "The real depths of nursing can only be made known through ideals, love, sympathy, knowledge and culture expressed through the practice of artistic procedures and relationships"[40, p. 476]. She wrote of curative and preventive nursing measures for physical and psychological patient needs. Her feeling for nursing was basically humanistic.

In the 1940s and 1950s, education in general took an abrupt turn away from the time-honored humanities to the rapidly emerging field of science. Nursing education and practice did also. Nursing began being defined as a science as well as an art. In 1947, Esther Lucille Brown defined the future role of the nurse as that of still recognizing and tending to the needs of the ill person, but in addition, "she will possess a body of scientific nursing knowledge which is based upon and keeps pace with general scientific advancement, and she will be able to apply this knowledge in meeting the nursing needs of a person and a community" [9, p. 73]. Miss Brown proved to be a far-sighted person, as the basic sciences began to take on a significant role in nursing education and practice in the 1950s, and have continued to do so today.

In the mid-1950s into the 1960s, nursing grappled with the problem of defining the role of the nurse within the framework of the health team. Medicine and nursing seemed to cross lines and merge at various points. Nursing leaders struggled with specific definitive guidelines for practice. Abdellah[1] published *Patient-Centered Approaches to Nursing* as a guide to specific patient-centered nursing. An effort was made to separate the nurse out of the total health team concept and examine her role, especially in patient interaction. The role was viewed as being a "unique process" in which the nurse identified, understood and met the patient's needs. Mental health principles became integrated into nursing, and an effort was directed toward total patient care. Nursing took on definition as a "significant, therapeutic, interpersonal process . . . [functioning] co-operatively with other human processes that make health possible for individuals in communities"[32, p. 16].

As time pushed into the 1970s, the nursing literature began utilizing terms such as *integrated mental-physical health care, problem-oriented nursing, preventive health care* and *individualized maintenance of behavioral integrity.* Many new terms and many old cliches have been used to define nursing along the long way, but just how far have we really come from Miss Nightingale's original premise, that the nurse's role is that of putting the patient "in the best condition" to enhance response and repair? Throughout the years, nursing has identified caring for the patient and his needs as the major focus of its endeavors. In an effort to keep up with vast scientific and medical advances, complexities of health technologies, increasing stresses of our fast-paced society and mountains of paperwork, however, the nurse has become a many-faceted, multidirectional, highly organized, systematized provider of care. Look at a modern coronary care unit. The patient's room is a bank of computers. The patient is monitored for all eventualities—lights flash, buzzers buzz, read-out tapes record all life functions and a television monitor records the entire scene for viewing at the nurse's station. The nurse can have an instant read-out of vital signs, the convenience of computer-controlled intravenous nourishment and adequate warning if any system fails. Still, something is missing.

Consider the average medical-surgical floor in the hospital. The patient is awakened at 7 a.m. to have his temperature taken with an electronic thermometer complete with digital read-out. The drip rate of his I.V. is monitored and controlled by an electronic eye. During the morning, the patient may have his bed made by an aide, his back rubbed by an L.P.N., his medications administered by an R.N. He may be transported by a volunteer to x-ray, radiation therapy or respiratory therapy where he is exposed to still more people, still more equipment. The patient soon learns that he is functioning within the hospital's routine and on its timetable, and that all his care must be completed by the magical hour of 11 a.m. Something is missing.

Somewhere amidst all that equipment, behind all that SOAP charting, among all those nursing care plans, there is a human being—the patient. Have we become so involved in keeping up with the fast-paced technology and science of nursing and the hospital organizational routines, that we have lost sight of the art, the caring *humanistic* side of nursing?

> The ever-increasing growth of health care technology demands a similar increase in the health care professional's ability to deal with the psychological concerns of the patient. For there is a real danger that the field of health care may become so enamored of its technology that the patient's emotional and psychological functioning will be increasingly ignored[4, p. ii].

It would appear that nursing is in need of a humanistic revolution, a return to the caring function of the nurse. It is our belief that a society weary of technology wants to put a stop to loss of identity and dehumanization, and that within our own profession, our patients desire a humane system of care that recognizes the humanity of us all as nursing priority number one.

THE NATURE OF NURSING

Nursing is a human service, always concerned directly or indirectly with people. A human service provides the necessities required by the individual to function to the fullest, mentally, physically and emotionally, and to realize his maximum potential for growth[8, p. xvi]. As a human service designed to work with people, nursing then becomes an interpersonal process that consists of a dynamic change-producing experience or series of experiences between people. In nursing, the goal of the process is positive change, i.e., improvement of the patient's physical and psychological status, identification and meeting of individualized patient needs, insight and learning on the part of both persons involved in the process. "Changes occur as a result of the impact of one individual on the other. To identify and be able to bring about change in a purposeful, enlightened, thoughtful manner is a nursing activity"[42, p. 8].

A major stumbling block to humanistic nursing seems to be inherent in the time-honored labels we apply to people and the perceptions these labels create. Each person is different, separate and original and must be recognized as one of a kind and related to as such, not be reduced to "the patient." The nurse-patient relationship is in actuality a person-to-person relationship. That is, two individuals share a dynamic experiential process while working toward some goal or objective. Each one maintains his individuality, while fostering his own personal growth toward self-actualization, and encouraging similar growth in the other person. The goal may be return to good health, preventive health teaching, emotional support or meeting any specific problem that is interfering with the patient's ability to function at optimum potential.

THE HUMANISTIC NURSE

Humanistic nursing is practiced by a self-actualized nurse who is the product of a humanistic education. In Chapter 1, we described the self-actualized person as one who is mature, competent, stable, flexible, interested and responsible, comfortable with himself and always in a "growing" state. We said this person possessed three outstanding qualities: empathy, respect (warmth) and genuineness. Let us now take a look at the qualities of the self-actualized humanistic nurse. ·

The humanistic nurse responds to the patient as a unique whole person. The process the nurse employs includes environmental changes conducive to goal-fulfillment and her own helping and assistive behavior "which enables the [patient] to fully experience, explore and resolve [his] problems and to become self-actualized"[17, p. 73].

In carrying out the process of interacting with the patient the nurse employs her humanistic qualities. She empathizes so that she might really understand what the patient feels and thereby recognize and comprehend his behavior. She "tunes in" to the patient in an attempt to assist him better in meeting his needs. She can accept his feelings and ideas, expressions and behaviors, as important to him and to his self-concept. Through this recognition and acceptance, the nurse can better define the patient s potential for and direction toward self-actualization. Her spontaneity of responsiveness, or genuineness, toward the patient further affirms her recognition of his worth. The humanistic nurse cares for and about people. Because she herself is self-actualized, she can allow for and foster self-actualization in others.

Two four-year-olds were playing when one asked the other, "What do you want to be when you grow up?" The second child answered, "I want to be *me,* only bigger and better." We all need the "me" in us to be recognized, respected and related to by others. This is the most significant role of the humanistic nurse —that among all the technology, I.V. bottles, time schedules, treatments and procedures, she sees the person inside the patient and relates to that person.

TRENDS IN NURSING EDUCATION

We believe that a humanistic form of nursing education can best facilitate the development of a humanistic nurse. From a historical perspective, many areas of nursing education are already humanistic and others are moving in that direction. In this section, we explore the history of nursing education with a special emphasis on tracing the development of humanistic trends. This review reveals that the transition of nursing education from hospitals to institutions of higher learning contributed greatly to the development of a humanistic approach.

Since its beginning in this country, nursing education has been and continues to be to a large extent dependent on nursing practice for providing student learning. Because of this close relationship, students have always participated as learners while providing health care services. Even today, the health service a student provides is a potential by-product of the education she receives, just as her education is a potential by-product of the health service she provides[2, p. 8]. As a result of this interdependent relationship and the early concept of nursing practice as being chiefly the delivery of technical skills, a large portion of nursing education has traditionally emphasized mastery of psychomotor skills as the major goal. Gradually, there has been a change in that emphasis, and the goals have broadened to include the cognitive and affective realms of learning.

Diploma School Nursing Education

From the establishment of the first nursing schools in this country in 1873 until the middle 1960s, the emphasis on student learning was dominated by the concept that the student must become proficient in technical tasks and procedures.

This was largely a result of the fact that hospital schools of nursing were originally established to serve a utilitarian purpose: they contributed to the cost efficiency of the hospital by ensuring hospitals of nursing staff at a low cost. These early schools were controlled by the hospitals and their primary aim was to provide service, not education. Little in the way of scientific principles or concepts was given as a background for teaching the functional tasks that a nurse must perform. This could be described as the era in which nursing education was dominated by one-sided striving for mastery of psychomotor skills or technical skills. Although the early nursing student's learning was based on experience, it definitely was not experiential education of a whole human being, since its focus did not include the affective and cognitive realms of development.

Initially, there were no special instructors to guide the learning. A student was part of the hospital staff, responsible to the head nurse and supervisors who directed her "training" in the proper performance of tasks and procedures. The head nurses and supervisors were usually students themselves, who were in the latter part of their training period. As the early nursing student learned her role through on-the-job training while being a full-time participant in the delivery of health care, her learning needs were secondary to the needs of the hospital. A student in a typical early hospital school of nursing received a preparatory three- to four-week course of classroom instruction, while at the same time working 25 to 30 hours a week. Classes were sporadic lectures offered by physicians. After these initial weeks, training took place strictly in the clinical setting and revolved around the needs of the hospital. As a result, the content of nursing education began and continued for many years to be disease-centered with emphasis on the medical therapeutic care plan. The education was clearly service-centered rather than student-centered or patient-centered. The individual needs of the learner were ignored, and the emotional needs of the patient were not considered. Nursing education was preparation only for a mechanical performance of tasks.

Another example of the early utilitarian function of nursing students was the practice of sending them without supervision into private homes to provide bedside care in exchange for a fee that the hospital collected. In these situations, the student not only saved money for the institution, she earned income for it. Often her practice was extended to increase the hospital's income[37].

Because of the financial asset of having the so-called training school provide free nursing service for the hospital, there was continued growth in their number from 1873 on, so that in 1910 there were over 1,000 such schools. During this time, nurses began expressing the need for further education. To accommodate this need, the training period was gradually lengthened from one or one and a half years to three years. This allowed for the extra content to be included, while maintaining the time deemed essential for on-the-job training.

From the beginning, the nature of the schools within institutions and the education offered raised questions as to whether the aim of the school was charitable service or education. In 1894, at the First Annual Convention of the American Society of Superintendents of Training Schools, leaders in nursing education stressed that the entire training program should be planned for educating the student and not for the convenience of the hospital nursing service, thus initiating the trend toward student-directed education.

In 1895, Linda Richards[22, p. 14] stressed the need for a more uniform curriculum of instruction and an elevation of standards for schools of nursing. Nursing education at this time varied widely among institutions. Some schools provided a course of lectures while others provided none, as they still believed nursing was merely a performance of routine tasks. Hence provision for cognitive education was considered unnecessary by a number of programs, and nurses were self-educated, if they were educated at all.

In spite of the opposition, recommendations were made to superintendents of training schools that a nursing curriculum should develop and maintain a cognitive format including medical, surgical, gynecological and obstetrical nursing for a designated period of time. Because the sizes and types of hospitals with training schools varied, the types of practical experience available to students differed. To account for these differences and to meet the format recommendations, students were frequently sent out "on affiliation" to neighboring hospitals to gain practical experience. Further problems were that the recommendations did not include identification of common objectives, and that instruction, when it was available for the format areas, continued to be provided by physicians. This meant that the content emphasis was still placed on medical diagnosis and treatment rather than on problems of the patient and nursing interventions. The learning situation remained rather undesirable. Class instruction, when provided, continued to be fit in around the twelve-hour working days. Students had little time to themselves. Recognition of this continuing utilitarian role led to recommendations in 1896 at the Third Annual Convention of Superintendents of Nursing Schools to shorten a student's work day from twelve hours to eight.

The fundamental conflict between nursing service and nursing education continued. At the turn of the century, a movement to alleviate the apprenticeship status of nursing education developed. The Johns Hopkins School of Nursing moved the instruction of nurses from the clinical setting of the hospital into the classroom. For the first time, nursing instructors were hired with full-time teaching responsibilities. Although the content of the education remained procedure-centered, this marked the beginning of the removal of the learning experience from the control of nursing service to being placed under the supervision of nurse educators. Unfortunately, this pattern did not become universal at this time, because it was considered too expensive for a hospital to hire nurses just to teach. In fact, as late as 1949, the majority of nursing programs did not recognize education as their primary focus, but rather viewed service to the hospital as an objective of equal significance to that of the education of students. Hospitals had developed a cheap source of good labor, which they were reluctant to eliminate. Instead, they continued to exploit it.

The year 1909 was a landmark for nursing education for two reasons. First, Adelaide Nutting[22, p. 17] emphasized the importance of including the mind as well as the body of the patient when providing nursing care. Although it was a big step to recommend educating the nurse to care for the whole patient, this psychological aspect was not generally included in the curricula of nursing schools, due to crowding of curriculum time by heavy work experience schedules. Second, the first school of nursing was established within a university setting. The initiator of this idea, Dr. Richard Olding Beard[22, p. 18], identified two equally desirable and significant purposes for nursing education. The first and primary purpose was to secure the highest and essentially symmetrical development of the physical, mental and spiritual potential of the individual. The second was to secure the greatest possible adaptation of the individual to the specific purposes toward which she wished to work. For the first time, the developmental needs of the individual learner became the primary educational focus; the vocational (task-oriented) phase was secondary. This was significant because the need for a broad foundation of knowledge on which to build the vocational phase of nursing education was stressed. Cognitive needs were again recognized as being important to the performance of competent nursing care.

This philosophy continued to contrast sharply with the concept generally held by those in nursing education that one learns best by doing. This idea was firmly supported by those institutions that had the most to gain from the service provided by students while they learned by doing. The conflict between the dual character of nursing schools to provide both education and service began to be recognized as a major problem. It was obvious that when the two were in conflict, meeting the needs of the service institution took precedence over meeting those of students.

A number of studies and surveys of nursing practice and education from 1923 through 1951 provided a barrage of criticism from many sources. This criticism eventually led to the development of an active program of accreditation of nursing programs by the National League for Nursing. Suggestions and recommendations that were set forth as a result led to progressive change. Slowly, nursing emerged as being more educationally oriented. The programs were shortened. Nursing educators gained control of student practice. Colleges began to be used extensively to provide courses in general educational subjects. What followed was the development of a wide divergence in the types of educational programs and in the educational objectives set for the kind of nurse the schools were striving to produce. Eventually there were three types of programs preparing registered nurses: diploma, associate degree and baccalaureate degree. As nursing schools became educationally oriented, students began to be used less and less for service functions. Economically, nursing programs became expensive for institutions to sponsor. Where once students were financial assets to a hospital, they became financial liabilities. In addition, the ANA position paper in 1965 supported the move of all nursing education into institutions of higher learning, thus establishing a goal of removing it from direct control by service institutions. As a result, recent history has seen the demise of the majority of diploma schools and an increase in both associate and baccalaureate degree education. Alas, the problem of divergence in the products of the three types of programs still plagues the profession.

Baccalaureate Nursing Education

Higher education goals. In order to meet the goals of professional higher education, early collegiate programs in nursing education were faced with a great need for change in their actual practice. Many of them had simply superimposed the hospital pattern of education on a liberal arts base without making an effort to integrate the broad liberal arts background into the nursing curriculum. Students in college-based programs frequently studied liberal arts for two years and then went into the three-year diploma hospital-based portion of the program. In 1922, Yale University School of Nursing took the lead in altering this approach in two ways. They included in the program content both the physical and psychological needs of the patient, and they changed their model from one using a physician-oriented case study to one using a patient-centered nursing care study. Yet as college and university programs continued to grow in number, their standards continued to vary. Not all adopted the approaches instituted by Yale. Many failed to require of nursing students the same standards they would require of students in other professional programs. They were still influenced by early service-oriented education.

Further study of nursing as a profession and nursing education as professional education was initiated. In 1953, Margaret Bridgman[22, p. 57] reaffirmed that basic education for nurses should be provided in colleges or universities. These programs were to include professional and profession-related general courses combining both the theoretical and technical aspects of nursing. Again, the need to meet the cognitive as well as the psychomotor learning needs of nursing students was stressed.

As the goals gradually encompassed the aims of professional education, Lambertson[22] examined the issues fully. The principles of professional education that she explored were essentially humanistic in nature. It is useful to review these principles here because their adaptation led to the current-day humanistic goals of nursing education. The trends and practices derived from them are discussed below.

1. *The goal of education is to teach students how to think critically so that they may continue to grow professionally and personally throughout their lives.*

Professional education prepares one to become a practitioner, not to be one. This is a major change from the task-oriented days of early nursing education that trained nurses to be proficient in procedures only. Today's nursing students are taught to think critically and to apply the nursing process in their care of patients.

2. *The curriculum represents the belief that education is an instrument of social change that reflects what the profession can or should be, rather than merely reflecting current practice.*

The discrepancy between education and service became more apparent with the introduction of a patient-centered approach[2]. It provided a humanistic organization to nursing content, an enormous change from the medically oriented content of early times. Patients were considered as individuals with unique problems that nursing could identify, and for which it could develop interventions. This approach introduced a new concept of patient care and provided a launching pad for new concepts of patient-oriented nursing that have permeated nursing education. The change, however, from task-oriented to patient-oriented care has been slow to occur. Thus, upon entering nursing practice, new graduates experience "reality shock"[21]. They have been taught nursing according to a whole-task or professional system of providing individualized patient care, while much of nursing practice is still organized on a bureaucratic functional care basis.

One premise in writing this book is that if nurses are to play a major role in defining nursing practice as patient-oriented and in developing ways to achieve this, they must be educated to be effective in bringing about change. To us, the ability to create or accept change has more to do with the personal growth and development of students toward self-actualization than with the development of their cognitive potential, although that, of course, is also a vital part of education.

3. *Educational objectives clearly state their goals of developing beginning competency levels for professional leadership.*

These objectives describe the behavior patterns or ways of reacting to situations that the school wishes the learner to develop. Nursing education is currently involved in developing more definitive beginning competency levels for graduates.

4. *The educational objectives reflect the faculty's philosophy of nursing practice.*

Obviously these now reflect a patient-centered, humanistic form.

5. *As the student progresses through the program, her objectives and those of the teacher become more similar.*

As a student matures through her educational experiences, she assumes increasing responsibility for identifying her needs as a learner. She also becomes more directive and achieves greater independence and responsibility for meeting those needs.

6. *Education is organized in an orderly progression from simple to the increasingly complex.*

A learning experience is not the content of the course or the teacher's methods of teaching. Learning takes place within the student; it is what he does that he learns. This implies that the learner is an active participant. A learning experience is conceived of as a sequence of planned activities, meaningful for the learner, through which he acquires new abilities to help him reach a goal[22, p. 64].

Today, the nursing student is no longer expected to perform as a full provider of care after one month's orientation. Education is student-centered, planned around her learning needs, not the service needs of the institution.

7. *Learning experiences should foster the opportunity to use scientific principles to solve professional problems.*

In nursing education, the student now experiences a planned clinical program in which she has the opportunity to apply the nursing process, a problem-solving technique, to develop solutions to problems. In the process of solving the problem, she applies her broad background of scientific principles learned from the physical, social and biological sciences. The importance of selecting a learning experience and guiding a student through it implies an emphasis on learning rather than on teaching.

Lambertson[22] incorporates in her discussion the humanistic idea that the teacher has the responsibility to guide learning in a conducive environment, one that facilitates student sharing rather than control. In support of this, she includes some propositions of learning theory by Nathaniel Cantor that he derived from clinical studies of personality [22, pp. 65–66].

a.   The pupil learns only what he is interested in learning.
b.   It is important that the pupil share in the development and management of the curriculum.
c.   Learning is integral.
d.   Learning depends upon wanting to learn.
e.   An individual learns best when he is free to create his own responses in a situation.
f.   Learning depends upon fixing the problem.
g.   Every pupil learns in his own way.
h.   Learning is largely an emotional experience.
i.   To learn is to change.

The implications of actually instituting this type of teaching philosophy in nursing education are considerable, and for the most part have not been accomplished. Nursing education at present remains teacher-centered. What is of significance is that this philosophy was first introduced into nursing education more than twenty years ago.

8. Effective professional education requires an appropriate connection between theory and practice.

A clinical learning experience in nursing provides a means for the student to assess the value of principles as well as to evaluate her own understanding of them in action.

9. The faculty of a professional program is responsible for all phases of the educational program.

Enforcement of this principle means that control of nursing education has to be separated from the service institutions in which it originated. Ramifications of this action, leading to the demise of most diploma programs, were discussed earlier.

10. Educational outcomes are dependent in a large way on a teacher's competence both as a teacher and as a professional practitioner.

A nurse educator has two areas of specialization: nursing and teaching. Competence in nursing is necessary, but not sufficient for skilled teaching. Nursing education now has the qualified faculty that it lacked originally. Recognition of the need for qualified faculty occurred in the early 1960s and led to federal government authorization for funding to support such faculty development. Since that time, nursing education has no longer been dependent on nursing service and physicians for teaching.

11. The teacher-student relationship demonstrates a humanistic philosophy of teaching and of the profession.

This relationship serves as a model and directly influences the student's relationship with her patients and her co-workers. As nursing students have been cognitively educated to meet the psychological needs of patients, nurse educators have been cognitively introduced to the importance of meeting the affective needs of students. The key to being able to do this lies within the teacher-student relationship. Although this principle recognizes learning as an emotional as well as an intellectual experience, nursing education began with an initial emphasis on intellectual learning, with some recognition that the learner's feelings influence what she learns and how she learns it. This principle needs to become implemented in the day-to-day process of nursing education.

12. Professional education requires a careful selection process to secure evidence of certain potentials for future achievement among applicants.

Lambertson[22] identified the need for systematic study in this area. Today, nurse educators in both associate and baccalaureate degree programs are involved in such research.

From this review, it is clear that the humanistic goals of nursing education have been adapted from those of broad general education, and that these have had far-reaching effects in various areas. A question that needs to be addressed, and will be later in this book, is the way in which these goals are being implemented.

Associate Nursing Education

Twenty-six years ago, a third type of nursing program, associate degree education, began to develop. This type of program was based on research in nursing practice and the existing nursing education system, which analyzed the implications of vocational and technical education for preparation for nursing. From this research, Montag[34, pp. 496–497] recommended that there be only two types of nurses, technical and professional, and that they be prepared totally in institutions of higher learning. The professional nurse was to be prepared in four-year university programs of nursing education, while the technical nurse was to be prepared in a new kind of program established within a junior college or community college system. This type of education was unique in that the school was totally independent of the hospital. It was to be two calendar years in length, with all clinical experiences carefully planned to coincide with classroom instruction. Cognitive learning became an integral, concurrent part of psychomotor learning. This was accomplished by using a method of teaching in the patient care setting that employed pre-clinical and post-clinical conferences, in which students and teachers could plan for and evaluate an educationally controlled clinical learning experience. This was one of the most significant innovations made in nursing education, and represented a major change from the affiliation-rotation on-the-job system of the 1940s. It is one that has now become commonplace throughout nursing education programs[34, pp. 500–501]. Theoretically, a dynamic group process occurs at the pre-clinical and post-clinical conference sessions[25, p. 503]. In reality, the conferences are usually teacher-directed, thus providing teacher-centered rather than student-centered learning.

The results of experimenting with this kind of program revealed that when a school had complete control of students, nurses could be trained at least as satisfactorily in two years as in three years, and under better conditions. While early nursing programs, even baccalaureate programs, taught little more than the techniques of medical therapy, associate degree programs insisted on teaching techniques of nursing practice. This has helped to bring nursing today closer to being truly professional than it has ever been in the past.

There have been numerous other contributions of associate degree programs to nursing education[34]. In associate degree programs, curriculum was no longer organized around the geography of the hospital, but around the nursing needs of patients. Almost all nursing programs are struggling with the identification of a theoretical framework to unify their curricula. Frequently, the framework used may be humanistic based on the theories of Maslow or Rogers. Still another contribution has been the use of behavioral terms to specify desired outcomes to learning. In addition, innovations of various educational technology have been introduced and adapted for individualizing the teaching. Some of these have been: closed-circuit television, audio-visual media and programmed instruction. They are now widely used in other nursing education programs.

A major premise of associate degree education[34] is that of preparing a student as a beginning practitioner who will upon graduation begin the process of becoming a fully competent practitioner. These programs do not send out into nursing practice a rigid, static, procedure- and task-oriented nurse, but rather a person who can solve problems and apply definite scientific principles safely in a variety of situations. The A.D. graduate's growth continues as she profits from work experience.

From this review, it is possible to see that associate degree education has been trend-setting during its history of a little more than 25 years. It has contributed to many areas of nursing education: establishment of goals, arrangement of curriculum and content, the process of education itself, and changes in the expectations of the graduates.

Continuing Trends

Today, the goal of nursing education is to prepare thinking, feeling graduates, well-rounded in psychomotor skills, who are able to function effectively in the modern world with its growing complexities. You could say that this goal is definitely humanistic, recognizing the nursing student as a whole person with physical, emotional and intellectual potential. The nursing profession is humanistic because it is patient-centered. It is common for a nursing curriculum to have a humanistic theoretical framework that provides organization and commonality to the integration of its program. Directed clinical learning experiences provide for both cognitive and psychomotor skill development. The helping process as learned from psychotherapy is being integrated throughout the curriculum, stressing the need to understand and respond to the behavior of every patient. These current trends all help contribute toward a humanistic foundation for nursing education.

In his book, Aspy[5] discusses applying an industrial production model to education in which there are three stages: input, process and outcome. These stages correspond to three questions for educators: Where do we begin? What do we do? Where do we finish? The humanistic foundation of nursing education can be viewed as part of the input section of this model.

The beginning point (input) of nursing education, as discussed, seems to be in good order. Examination of the graduates (outcome), however, indicates a need for improvement elsewhere in the system. The graduates have thus far been unable to initiate the kind of changes in nursing practice that would enable them to provide the humanistic, individualized care that their education is preparing them to provide. Nurses, even a year after graduation, are still unable to apply their knowledge and are unable to make appropriate changes in the system to make it more patient-centered. Kramer and Schmalenberg[21] offer some suggestions for the new graduate to use in resolving the conflict she experiences between her personal values that have developed during her education and the values of the workplace. Yet when the conflict is resolved, nursing practice remains unchanged.

That this change is necessary is not in question. Toffler[41] says that the more we learn about stress and tension, the more we realize that resistance to it is what may determine whether or not people get well, stay well or become ill. Several studies[10; 33] have shown that experimental nursing care that is focused on giving information, instruction or psychological support has improved patient welfare, as evidenced by shortened length of hospital stay and decreased amount of pain medication needed after surgery. The studies indicate that supportive nursing activities reduce stress and tension in patients, and because of this reduction, these patients demonstrated more satisfaction and expressed fewer complaints than those with a higher level of anxiety.

It becomes clear that the practice of nursing must foster the kind of interpersonal process that provides caring and humanizes both client and nurse. If it is to do this, a humanistic, self-actualizing, responsible nurse is needed. Examining the process of nursing education may provide clues as to why this is not happening.

Aspy[5] suggests that educators look at the day-to-day process of education and assess how effective it is in fostering the growth of students toward self-actualization. Process, according to Aspy, refers to the interpersonal interactions that occur during the school day. It reveals what actually happens instead of what we wish would happen. It is by looking at the process that we see what is actually happening in day-to-day nursing education.

Epstein[16, pp. 3-4] states that the process of nursing education persists in being rigid. She says that as long as practitioners of a profession are educated in situations and by methods that encourage rigidity, and as long as they ignore human relations education, the profession is stacking the deck against itself. It is fostering its own rigidity to change. She continues by saying that this does not mean that there are not a lot of students who appear perfectly willing to continue their passive, conformist roles. They have learned this role well throughout their experience in elementary and secondary schools. The students are not satisfied and content; they are passive and conforming. It is this learned response that dulls creativity and breeds resignation. No wonder our graduates cannot make changes.

Currently, the process of nursing education is not only rigid, it is teacher-centered. Classroom discussion is a myth[16]. No such thing exists. What happens is that the teacher talks with five or six students while the rest listen. Other classroom procedures include the lecture, during which the teacher tells what she feels is important for the learner to know. Small group discussions by students in pre-clinical and post-clinical conferences tend to be teacher-centered, teacher-led discussions with interaction occurring between the teacher and one student at a time. Interaction among students is stifled and at a minimum.

It is easy to say that the process of nursing education must be changed. It must be made more humanistic. The student must be allowed to become an active participant in the process of learning. The issue then raised is how to accomplish this. McLuhan and Fiore[26, p. 8] say that social interactions (the medium), not the subject matter (the content), have the most impact. If we accept this premise, nurse educators need to become facilitators of processes that foster student interaction. They must also model empathy, respect, warmth and genuineness to create an environment that is conducive to the total growth of students.

Nurse educators are becoming aware of this need to change. They are looking for ways to implement their humanistic objectives within the learning process and to make the process congruent with their end goals. Current nursing literature reveals an increased focus on the process of learning. Many of the models being developed are experiential and provide for the learning needs of the whole student. They enhance dynamic interaction integrating all three realms of learning. Some examples of the types of models being developed in undergraduate nursing programs are as follows: (1) simulation experiences[24] are being utilized for teaching patient assessment; (2) instructional drama[23] has minimized intellectualization when teaching how to care for and respond to a dying patient; (3) simulation gaming[12], a combination of both simulation and games, has been used to create an experiential situation that mimics processes or conditions that actually occur; (4) videotaping a student's clinical experiences in the hospital[19] provides a dynamic approach to teaching better patient care by enhancing the student's ability to evaluate and improve her own clinical performance; (5) a group approach to applying research techniques to nursing practice[36] provides a personal experience with doing research; (6) student-centered group process in pre-clinical and post-clinical conferences[20] is described as fostering positive dynamic interaction among students; (7) Epstein[16] proposes several techniques and exercises such as "census taking" and small task groups for involving students totally in both the planning and the process stages of education; and (8) Cowart[14] teaches a course entitled "Legislative Influences on Health Care" in which she uses simulated committee meetings, experiential activities within the bureaucratic and private sectors for which students record their interactions and reactions in a two-part log, doing research in an area of special interest and developing this study project into a draft of a bill, and independent study of a student-selected topic or legislative issue that is presented in seminar discussion. The discussions of each of these models have in common a description of positive effects on the learning process. Empirical observation revealed growth-producing interaction in cognitive, affective and psychomotor learning.

These examples indicate that nursing education is beginning to take up the challenge of providing a humanistic process within its educational system. Hopefully, this trend will lead to the education of humanistic self-actualizing nurses who can accomplish satisfactory changes in professional practice.

Nurse educators have an added responsibility beyond establishing these kinds of models and collecting empirical evidence that shows these models to be effective in promoting humanistic learning. They need to document through systematic research the effect that humanizing the process has on both the day-to-day education of nursing students and on the development of a humanized nursing practice.

REFERENCES

1. Abdellah, F.; Martin, A.; Beland, I.; and Matheney, R. *New Directions in Patient-Centered Nursing*. New York: Macmillan, 1973.
2. Abdellah, F.; Martin, A.; Beland, I.; and Matheney, R. *Patient-Centered Approaches to Nursing*. New York: Macmillan, 1960.
3. Altman, S. *Present and Future Supply of Registered Nurses*. Rockville, Md.: U.S. Department of Health, Education and Welfare, DHEW publication No. (NIH), pp. 72–134, 1971.
4. Anthony, W., and Carkhuff, R. *The Art of Health Care*. Amherst, Mass.: Human Resource Development Press, 1976.
5. Aspy, D. *Toward a Technology for Humanizing Education*. Champaign, Ill. Research Press, 1972.
6. Bensman, P. Have we lost sight of the A.D. philosophy? *Nursing Outlook* 25:511–513, 1977.
7. Beverly, L., and Junker, M. The A.D. nurse: Prepared to be prepared. *Nursing Outlook* 25:514–518, 1977.
8. Brill, N. *Team-work: Working Together in the Human Services*. New York: Lippincott, 1976.
9. Brown, E. L. *Nursing for the Future*. New York: Russell Sage, 1948.
10. Chapman, J. Effect of different nursing approaches on psychological and physiological responses. *Nursing Research Report* 5(1):1–4, 1970.
11. Chapman, J., and Chapman, H. *Behavior and Health Care: A Humanistic Helping Process*. St. Louis: Mosby, 1975.
12. Clark, C. Simulation gaming: A new teaching strategy in nursing education. *Nurse Educator* 1(4):4–9, 1976.
13. Corcoran, S. Should a service setting be used as a learning laboratory? *Nursing Outlook* 25:771–776, 1977.
14. Cowart, M. Teaching the legislative process. *Nursing Outlook* 25:777–780, 1977.
15. deTornyay, R. Changing student relationships, roles, and responsibilities. *Nursing Outlook* 25:188–193, 1977
16. Epstein, C. *Effective Interaction in Contemporary Nursing*. Englewood Cliffs, N.J.: Prentice-Hall, 1974.
17. Haber, J.; Leach, A.; Schudy, S.; and Sidealeau, B. *Comprehensive Psychiatric Nursing*. New York: McGraw-Hill, 1978.
18. Henderson, V., and Nite, G. *Principles and Practice of Nursing*. New York: Macmillan, 1978.
19. Holland, J. Videotaping clinical experience. *Nursing Outlook* 25:337–338, 1977.
20. King, V. A confluent approach to nursing education through group process. *Nurse Educator* 3(3):20–25, 1978.
21. Kramer, M., and Schmalenberg, C. *Path to Biculturalism*. Wakefield, Mass.: Contemporary Publishing, 1977.
22. Lambertson, E. *Education for Nursing Leadership*. Philadelphia: Lippincott, 1958.
23. Lewis, F. A time to live and a time to die. *Nursing Outlook* 25:762–765, 1977.

24. Lincoln, R.; Layton, J.; and Holdman, H. Using simulated patients to teach assessment. *Nursing Outlook* 26:316–320, 1978.
25. Martin, B., and McAdory, D. Are A.D. clinical experiences adequate? *Nursing Outlook* 25:502–505, 1977.
26. McLuhan, M., and Fiore, Q. *The Medium is the Massage.* New York: Random House, 1967.
27. Michelmore, E. Distinguishing between AD and BS education. *Nursing Outlook* 25:506–510, 1977.
28. Mitchell, P. *Concepts Basic to Nursing* (2nd ed.). New York: McGraw-Hill, 1977.
29. Nightingale, F. *Notes on Nursing, What It Is and What It Is Not.* (Re-publication of first American edition published by D. Appleton & Co., 1860.) New York: Dover, 1969.
30. Orem, D., and Parkee, K. *Nursing Content in Preservice Nursing Curriculum.* Washington, D.C.: Catholic University Press, 1964.
31. Partridge, K. Nursing values in a changing society. *Nursing Outlook* 26:356–360, 1978.
32. Peplau, H. *Interpersonal Relations in Nursing.* New York: Putnam, 1952.
33. Putt, A. One experiment in nursing adults with peptic ulcers. *Nursing Research* 19:484–494, 1970.
34. Rines, A. Associate degree education: History, development, and rationale. *Nursing Outlook,* 25:496–501, 1977.
35. Rines, A., and Montag, M. *Nursing Concepts and Nursing Care.* New York: Wiley, 1976.
36. Schare, B. An undergraduate research experience. *Nursing Outlook* 25:178–180, 1977.
37. Schweer, J., and Gebbie, K. *Creative Teaching in Clinical Nursing.* St. Louis: Mosby, 1976.
38. Smoyak, S. Teaching as coaching. *Nursing Outlook* 26:361–363, 1978.
39. Stevens, B. The teaching-learning process. *Nurse Educator* 1(1):9;12–15;18–20, 1976.
40. Taylor, E. Of what is the nature of nursing? *American Journal of Nursing* 34:476, 1934.
41. Toffler, A. *Future Shock.* New York: Random House, 1970.
42. Travelbee, J. *Interpersonal Aspects of Nursing.* Philadelphia: Davis, 1971.

CHAPTER 3

A Combined Learning Theory

In the previous chapters we reviewed and discussed humanistic philosophy and the significance of applying it to nursing education. We observed that present philosophies and objectives in nursing education are basically humanistic in orientation. On taking a closer look, however, it is clear that the day-to-day process of nursing education needs to be humanized in order to implement these objectives. What is needed is the selection of a learning theory that will provide a humanistic approach in nursing education.

The learning theory that we have selected and with which we have worked has several components. It combines the principles of Gestalt therapy, confluent education and group process. These components will be reviewed and discussed individually and as an integrated whole.

Much of the work that has been done in confluent education is based on the theory of Gestalt therapy; their interrelationships are numerous and complex, based largely on the concept that Gestalt therapy is also a theory of learning.

PHILOSOPHY OF GESTALT THERAPY

Gestalt therapy includes a philosophy of how human growth and development occur, as well as a methodology for facilitating them. In Gestalt therapy, the concept of holism is essential to the development of human potential. Even the word *gestalt,* when translated, means "a whole." Gestalt theorists believe that the introduction of this concept into our current age is a necessity because we have lost an awareness of our wholeness, and the complex union of our body, mind and emotions. Instead, we have become accustomed to thinking of ourselves as being divided into the separate entities—mind, body and feelings. It is common to think of our mind and body as being totally unrelated to our feelings—often with our mind being in control of our feelings. Gestalt therapy unifies this division.

The mind does not cause the body to operate, nor the body the mind; to conceive of things in that way is to emphasize their separateness. Instead, the pounding of our heart, our excitement, and the concurrent anxiety are manifestations of the same occurrence, like heat and light from the sun. Holistically, we cannot understand ourselves by summing our understanding of our heart, our brain, our nervous system, our limbs, our circulatory system. We are not simply an accumulation of functions[17, p. 6].

Thus, the whole of a person is not only greater than any one individual part, but it is greater than the sum of all parts. It is impossible to understand an isolated element of a person without considering the whole.

Gestalt therapy goes even beyond the holistic concept of a person as an individual, to that of a person being at one with the environment. It unites the functioning of body, thought and feelings with environment into an integrated whole. "I and the universe are one. All of me and all of the infinity of activities and energy around me, people and things, all of them together are one figure. Nothing is excluded"[17, p. 226]. The ultimate gestalt is a beginning awareness of the immensity of the extent of our interaction with everything else and experiencing this to the depths of our being, leaving nothing out[17, p. 227].

This is accomplished through increasing one's ability to be aware of and in touch with oneself—emotions, thoughts and sense of physical being. The person who experiences living in this manner is creative, self-actualizing, responsible, flexible and open to change.

According to Gestalt philosophy, there are certain principles of biological structure and functioning that can be observed in natural behavior. The principles we have selected to highlight are: (1) self-regulation of the organism, (2) formation and destruction of gestalts, (3) support functions of the organism and its environment field, (4) the self, (5) modes of the self, (6) polarities, or opposites in life, (7) awareness of self and its relationship to the universe, (8) responsibility and (9) completing or concluding the process of gestalt formation. The dynamics of these principles provide insight into the creative process of living. A description of these principles tends to make them appear static, but they are not; they are involved in continuous dynamic interplay and integration, organizing the process of living. Unfortunately, talking about these structures is inadequate. One needs to experience them to develop a feeling for them and grasp them fully. Thus we have included some examples of these principles in action. Hopefully, they will provide a little of the experiential flavor necessary to gain an understanding of them.

Self-Regulation of the Organism

If let alone, an organism will spontaneously regulate itself in all areas of function —appetite, sexuality, culture, learning and so forth. This is in line with some advice from Tao philosophy, "stand out of the way"[24, p. 291]. Essential to this principle of self-regulation is the need for an organism to be aware of its balance and imbalances and what is needed to correct the imbalances.

The concept of self-regulation does not suggest or ensure the satisfaction of the needs of an organism. It only implies that, if allowed, organisms will do their best to regulate themselves. Given their own capabilities and the resources of the environment, organisms will pick and choose what they need to support themselves. They will synthesize those parts of what is available (such as food, ideas and values) that they like and find useful, and assimilate them, make them part of themselves.

According to Latner[17, p. 16], organismic self-regulation is an ongoing process of distinguishing needs, determining the means by which they can be satisfied and organizing them into a cohesive whole (a gestalt) of understanding and activity, then carrying out that activity to its satisfying conclusion of need fulfillment. When the organism meets its need, thereby restoring its balance, the united functioning, the gestalt, that occurs as a result of the imbalance will disappear. This process occurs over and over throughout the life span of the organism.

Another dimension to this principle is that the organism functions with a prudence born of its needs and their fulfillment[17, p. 17]. In other words, the organism will demonstrate wisdom and economy in its behavior. It will not be greedy unless its ability to regulate itself has been disturbed. While wild animals kill only for food and not for pleasure, this may not be true for humans and domesticated animals. Their ability for regulation can become disturbed by lack of awareness.

Formation and Destruction of Gestalts

This is the key way in which the process of organismic self-regulation works. A gestalt is a whole—a configuration, a pattern, a focus of attention and activity that is developed to fulfill a need. That which comes into focus in order to satisfy the need is called the figure. That which does not become part of the focus remains the background. Gratification of a need results in its disappearance, and leads to fading of the gestalt into the background[17, pp. 26-32]. The gestalt formation is not actually destroyed, it is used in the future to help form another gestalt. Organismic regulation depends on the continual formation and destruction of gestalts. Another way of saying this is that a gestalt is based on our needs, it is what our self-regulation requires.

An example of gestalt formation and destruction[19, p. 47] frequently offered is that of a person reading a book, and suddenly becoming thirsty. As thirst becomes a priority need, a gestalt is formed around meeting this need. The person puts down the book, goes into the kitchen, pours a glass of water, drinks it and returns to reading. There may have been many possibilities in the person's environment, but the focus of his attention and activity (his gestalt) organized around thirst. Thirst became the focus or the figure, the rest of the environment remained in the background. Living is seen as a continual process of completing gestalts, or wholes.

Another aspect that bears mentioning is that of split gestalts[17, pp. 32-34]. We have all probably had the experience of doing many things at once: listening to the radio while cooking or sewing, or carrying on several other activities. In this situation, our energies are split betwen two or more gestalts. We may end up trying to do both or several if we cannot make a priority decision. This can create weak diffuse gestalts that tend to lack a sense of closure and the rewarding satisfaction that accompanies completion of a strong, unified single gestalt.

Support Functions of the Organism and Its Environment Field

"Every organism needs an environment to exchange essential substance—air, love"[22, p. 5]. The organism is an intrinsic part of the environment, embedded in it, its life dependent on it. Just as the sensory and motor systems of an organism can reach out to its environment, the reverse is also true: an environment can reach out and demand attention from an organism. Healthy functioning, the realization of an organism's full potential, requires environmental support. If the support is insufficient, the organism will be unable to meet all of its needs; the absence of support may be fatal for the organism.

Growth and maturity lend another dimension to this concept[17. pp. 54-56]. Maturity means moving away from environmental support toward self-support. While environmental support is essential, a person's health is undermined if he does not learn to use his own resources to fulfill his needs. If he continues to rely on other aspects of the environment to do for him what he can do for himself, he can impair the process of his gestalt formations by losing the distinction between himself and the environment.

All people need support both from within and from without. Each person finds for himself a suitable balance of self-supports and environmental supports. Unfortunately, some people have inadequate self-support systems and tend to lean heavily on environmental supports. This can be a big problem. There is a failure to develop responsibility for oneself. The dependent individual can become hurt, disappointed or shattered when the person to whom he gives this power fails to live up to expectations[29, p. 40].

The Self

This is the term in Gestalt therapy that means the whole person. Although some of the vocabulary (id, ego, self) was devised by Freud, these terms are used in ways particular to Gestalt therapy. Latner[17, pp. 56-60] says that in Gestalt therapy, personality and its organization refer to the figure (gestalt) of the individual as he is known over a period of time. It is manifested differently in different situations, like a hand that is closed into a fist, then open, giving, then curved around another hand. Any one of these hands by itself might be healthy or deformed, but all together they are a person's hand in various situations and at different times. Similarly, the various facets of the self are elements of a process that must be considered as a whole. The fundamental characteristic of the self is gestalt formation and destruction, working for the existence and growth of the organism.

Modes of the Self

Depending on the requirements of a situation, the self has different modes or styles of functioning: the id mode and the ego mode[17, pp. 60-65]. The id is the functioning of the self at the opposite pole from the ego. Where the id mode is relaxed and passive, the ego mode is deliberate, willful and active. The id mode of functioning occurs when one responds automatically. In this mode, the self processes go on seemingly without explicit direction from the self. The ego mode of functioning occurs when the person identifies what is of interest to him, meets his needs and discards what is uninteresting. In this mode, the individual is actively involved, consciously identifying and making decisions, dividing the environment into parts with which the gestalt is identified and parts from which it is alienated. The id and ego styles of functioning seldom occur in their pure form. Behavior is usually composed of elements of both. The relative importance of each style is related to the type of activity a person is engaged in and that individual's own personal style.

Polarities

Gestalt formation ends with the building of a unified whole of meaning and activity that results in satisfying an organism's needs[17, pp. 41-45, 180-183]. In determining which elements to combine into workable wholes, however, one must know what is available. This occurs through the process of differentiating what is available into opposites. Life is made up of polar extremes, for example, work/play, happy/sad, good/bad, likes/dislikes, friends/enemies. The relationship of opposites is such that the existence of one necessarily requires the existence of the other. In the process of Gestalt formation and destruction, it is essential that a person consider and integrate the opposite poles into the process. The result is synthesis built on the integration of the two, which meets the needs of the organism. The gestalt disappears and balance is restored between the organism and the environment.

Recognition of polarities within the client by the therapist is essential in Gestalt therapy. Once the client becomes aware of the polarities, it is equally important not to stop the process of gestalt formation, but to complete the synthesis stage by building a solution that integrates the two extremes and meets the needs of the client.

Awareness of Self and Its Relationship to the Universe

The most essential aspect to healthy functioning is awareness, the ability to apprehend with the full use of one's senses the world, both inside and outside oneself. Being in the present ensures the existence of the gestalt formation process in all its aspects. To be here and now means to allow that process to come about and work itself through to closure and satisfaction. It is necessary to know and be aware of oneself in order to determine one's needs, and to be aware of the pertinent parts of the environment available for use in meeting them. The process of gestalt formation cannot go on without an individual's participation in it. As a person can deal only with what he knows, this participation is only possible if the person is aware and in touch with himself and the outer world.

Responsibility

A person is responsible if he is aware of what is happening to him[24, pp. 26-27]. For a person to take responsibility means to accept his existence as it occurs. He identifies with his acts, impulses and feelings, accepting all of what he does as his. A person is responsible for his feelings not because he caused them to be, but because they constitute his existence at any moment in time. Always speaking from "I" assists an individual toward this ownership. An example of this would be to say, "I am angry . . ." rather than to shift the responsibility on to someone else: "You make me angry." If one becomes aware of what is going on in one's life, one can assume responsibility for whether it shall continue or cease to exist. This is different from the concept of responsibility that has at its center the notion of moral blame.

Concluding the Process

The completion of the gestalt is the creation of knowledge, or truth pertinent to a particular situation. Latner[17, p. 80] says this is learning, growing, discovering; it is making personal knowledge meaningful and useful. A quote from Perls [23, p. 18] expands this notion: "When we discover, we uncover our own ability, our own eyes, in order to find our potential, to see what is going on, to discover how we can enlarge our lives, to find means at our disposal that will let us cope with a difficult situation." A person gains from finding his own solutions. He learns to depend on himself for gratification of the whole hierarchy of his needs. He is not totally independent, but has what he needs to direct and control his own life and solve his own problems. There are times when he may repeat new solutions until he has thoroughly mastered them. This is known as digesting or assimilating the gestalt. Frequently, a child will do this when he learns something new.

As a new gestalt fades away it evolves into a feeling of peace and satisfaction. The organism is in balance. There is no need to fulfill, no surplus to discharge, no present business at hand. This is called a state of indifference or general openness without awareness of anything in particular. Each of us has probably experienced this, perhaps after completing some project in which we have been wholeheartedly involved.

In thinking about behavior we can see that these introductory descriptions of Gestalt principles may not seem to explain every situation. This is because they are only a simple and brief introduction to the Gestalt philosophy of human behavior. These basic principles, however, which describe the process of human growth and the realization of human potential, are crucial to our combined learning theory.

METHODOLOGY OF GESTALT THERAPY

Gestalt therapy methodology consists of a variety of techniques that are based on Gestalt principles. These techniques are used both to facilitate human growth and development and to restore healthy behavior. Fundamental is the belief that the process of gestalt formation and destruction is common to all human beings, and that the adequate functioning of this process is an essential aspect of healthy behavior. If this process is working effectively, it can enable a person to find positive solutions to dilemmas and challenges.

"Health is possessing the ability to deal successfully with any situation we encounter now, and success is the satisfactory resolution of situations according to the dialectic of gestalt formation and destruction . . . . To be able to be grounded in this process and live with it is maturity"[17]. Growth is the continual reorganization of ourselves and our environment. Gestalt process makes possible the perpetual creative adjustments to life that are part of healthy living. In fact, the more developed one's gestalt process is, the more able one is to develop one's potential for becoming self-actualizing. The ultimate goal of Gestalt therapy is to enhance the spontaneous and autonomous activity of an individual's gestalt process.

An earlier discussion reviewed the dominant role that awareness plays in the proper functioning of this process. Based on this central principle is the concept that diminished awareness is the primary cause of interference with the formation of productive gestalts[17]. When awareness, which is a person's experience of what is happening to him, becomes diminished, the gestalt process becomes weak. A lack of awareness precipitates the malfunctioning of the process and allows the malfunction to continue. Overcoming this lack of awareness forms the focal point of Gestalt therapy and is the key to either enhancing or restoring the independent and spontaneous activity of an individual's gestalt process. "In Gestalt therapy, we do this by attending to how we go about living our lives—how we function in the world, and how we can function more in tune with our nature"[17, p. 153]. A person first inquires into the ways in which he presently deals with the problems he faces in order to increase his awareness of this; then he carefully develops an experimental approach toward changing his functioning to make it more satisfying to him.

If people continue functioning with diminished awareness, unaware of their disproportionate dependency on their environment, their bending to outside control and their manipulative and resistive behavior, they are unable to bring about change and correct their malfunctioning.

Awareness

Gestalt therapy is sometimes defined as awareness training. An individual is helped to be aware of the here and now in feeling and sensory terms; not in terms of why he is behaving so, but rather in terms of what he is doing (physical action) and how he is experiencing it (i.e., feeling angry, happy, sad) and the bodily sensing of tightened muscles, clenched teeth, crying, smiling, relaxed muscles, and so forth.

Subjective and objective knowing are combined to facilitate awareness. From empiricism comes the idea of observation. For example[19, p. 49], a therapist observes a client grinding his teeth (objective knowing). Instead of measuring, analyzing and fitting the observation into a theoretical framework, and abstracting and moving the observation away from the current situation, however, the therapist asks the client to integrate the clenched teeth into his own awareness (subjective knowing). This does not mean he points out the observation to the client, but rather he asks the client, "Are you aware of what your teeth are doing?" The concern lies not with the therapist's awareness, but rather with the client's awareness. The client's awareness, however, might not emerge without the therapist's observations. In education, the teacher may need to facilitate a student's awareness of his strengths and weaknesses in this same nonjudgmental manner.

The techniques in Gestalt therapy are geared first toward increasing an individual's awareness through uncovering his present functioning, and second, toward discovering more adequate ways in which he can function. The techniques focus on helping a person get to know himself and his environment, to be aware of the present and be totally in it. When this occurs, the self is ensured of working as it is meant to work. The self is the person, the accumulation of his experiences, heredity and predispositions. As a person's awareness is enlarged, the self comes closer to fullness and adequacy. The person comes in touch with areas with which he is unable to deal satisfactorily and discovers resources within himself that assist him to develop new solutions to meet both his needs and those of his environment in a more satisfactory way[17, pp. 56-60; 153-154].

Awareness Skills

In order to develop and maintain awareness, an individual needs to sharpen various skills. Some of these skills are discrimination, contact, manipulation, expression of emotion and recognition of resistances. Because each is an important part of awareness, each will be reviewed individually.

Discrimination The skill of discrimination is to know what is us and what is not, what is the past and what is the present, what is pertinent to our needs and what is not[17, pp. 174-180].

Contact "Contact refers literally to the nature and quality of the way we are in touch with ourselves, our environment and the processes that relate them"[17, p. 65]. Contact is being able to reach out to another person, to our environment, to our inner self and to our opposite poles in order to make relevant use of our own resources and those in our environment to meet our needs. Successfully meeting a need and solving a problem provides support for increasing and expanding the skill of making contact. Each successful contact that fulfills a need becomes support for future contact and future gestalt formation.

Manipulation Manipulation—or rather, a person's manipulative faculties—is organized by the motor system. These faculties permit the individual to make changes in his environment or in his relationship to it. This is what allows the individual and his environment to make contact with each other and to interact in a process of mutual accommodation that in Gestalt therapy is called creative adjustment. The person who is thirsty is able to manipulate himself and the environment in order to satisfy his thirst[17, pp. 21-22].

Expressing Emotions "An emotion is a focusing of our excitement in such a way that our experiences have meaning. Emotions are the meaning of our experience. Gestalt therapy encourages experiencing and expressing intense emotions because they make our existence understandable and satisfying"[17, p. 173]. If a person shies away from making contact with his feelings he diminishes his life. Although feelings may be threatening to a person, according to Gestalt therapy staying in touch with the elements of one's experience acts to strengthen the self, not to destroy it. This does not mean spewing out emotions for the sake of ventilation. Rather, it means being in touch with feelings that are intrinsic to one's experience,

and expressing them so that they become part of the mix out of which new solutions emerge.

Resistance. Resistance impedes growth. A person needs help in recognizing his
resistance when it occurs. It is the ego mode's restraint on free functioning because a person has lost track of what he is trying to do or because he feels endan-
gered. Being in touch with one's resistances allows one the choice of whether or
not to try another way to behave. Having the choice permits responsibility for
oneself. Responsible behavior is essential for one to develop self-actualizing attributes[17, pp. 186-192].

Developing awareness is accomplished by helping a person increase his skills in
all of the above areas. This is the first step in the process of growth toward self-
actualization.

Acceptance and Integration

The process of living is one of continual change and growth. To be part of that
process requires awareness plus acceptance of the awareness. Gestalt therapy not
only facilitates development of awareness but helps one accept and integrate it.
A person is helped to face the facts of his life that he has hidden from himself,
to reclaim and integrate them as part of his whole self[17, pp. 49-50]. "Change
occurs when one becomes what he is, not when he tries to become what he is
not"[3, p. 77]. This is a paradoxical theory of change. Change does not take
place through a coercive attempt by an individual or another person to change
him, but it can and does take place if a person is able to take the time and effort
to be what he is and to be fully aware of his current positions. When a person becomes aware of and accepts what makes up his existence at this moment in his
life, he makes change possible. This ultimately makes growth possible.

Gestalt therapy does not offer a person solutions to his problems, because solutions that are not arrived at out of conflict and by the individual involved are unable to meet the person's real needs. They also tend to foster dependency. Instead,
the Gestalt therapist uses techniques that help the individual become aware of
and contact his own needs and resources. This is the first step toward being able
to create one's own solutions to problems.

Gestalt Therapy Techniques

There are as many techniques used in Gestalt therapy as there are therapists.
Each therapist has his own style because he has assimilated the principles and
developed a style of implementing them. Techniques arise out of the needs of
situations, and are not fixed by prior practices. Nonetheless, some methods have

come into common use and form the basis for the many variations in techniques. These will be reviewed briefly.

They include (1) role playing by an individual of his fantasy, dreams or memory; (2) using immediacy (processing what is happening right here and now); (3) changing language from using the word "it" to using the word "I" (as a way to assume responsibility for behavior and ownership of feelings); (4) learning how to talk with someone rather than at or about them; (5) processing awareness of bodily sensations; (6) staying with verbalizing feelings until they become understood and integrated. Examples of these techniques, some of which are from literature about Gestalt therapy, and others that are from writings about confluent education, provide illustration.

Role playing. Role playing in Gestalt therapy is probably the most difficult method to understand. It differs from the usual concept of role playing in which more than one person participates. In Gestalt therapy, the client himself imagines and acts out all the parts in a situation. The therapist concentrates on *how* the client is acting now, *not* on *why* he is acting that way. This technique can be used in a variety of ways to help a person understand himself, his relationships, his dreams, his fantasy and his reality.

Perls developed a special chair technique for role playing[22, p. 121]. The client sits on the "hot-seat" facing an empty chair onto which he projects his many selves. By using this technique, the opposing forces (poles) within a person can talk with each other, have it out with each other, forgive each other, compromise or at least come to know each other[16, p. 8].

This technique is used in a similar manner to clarify relationships between people, i.e., a student and a patient or a student and a staff member. A person with a problem imagines someone sitting opposite him in the other chair. He carries on a conversation with that person, bringing the situation or problem with which they are dealing into the here and now. He speaks to that person and expresses what he wants to say and then takes the role of the other person and responds.

Dreams can also be treated in this manner to gain self-awareness. The message in the dream, however, is clarified not by analyzing it but by reliving it. "Each person and each thing in the dream is some aspect of the dreamer. By role playing the people in the dream, the objects in the dream or even a fragment, the existential message that the dream holds can be unlocked . . ."[16, pp. 9–10].

In Gestalt therapy one's gestures, movements, feelings, speech, posture, expressions and interaction with reality are available to be worked with. A Gestalt therapist works in the present dealing with what is in front of him, the surface of behavior, helping a client become aware of this part of himself. He does not deal with the deep-seated unconscious, but with the obviousness of present functionings related through the role playing. By increasing awareness, a person is more in contact with the world because discovering additional aspects of the self and its functioning opens him to new experiences and new interactions with the world.

Variations of this technique have been used successfully in a variety of educational settings[7].

Immediacy. Immediacy is an important skill that is used to help the client understand himself and the world from a more objective point of view. He learns that it can promote growth both to be told how he is being experienced, and to tell another how he is experiencing[8, pp. 170-180]. This skill is used to handle transference when it occurs. If the patient attempts to deal with the therapist as though the therapist is the patient's parent, the therapist does not assume that role but remains himself. He helps the patient become aware of what is happening currently between himself and the therapist, i.e., that he is unable to distinguish between the fantasy of his parent and the reality of the therapist. The transference itself becomes an issue for exploration through immediacy.

> Therapist: I sense from what you have been telling me that you do not really trust me, that you cannot believe that I would want to help you.
> Client: Well, you sure listen to me a lot which no one else ever does, but no one really cares enough about me to want to help me. I'm not sure you do either.

In an educational setting, the teacher may need to process the relationship between himself and a student or students—what is going on here and how—before proceeding on to other aspects of learning.

Language changes. Language changes can be important in helping people to assume responsibility for their ideas, attitudes, opinions and feelings. The language shift usually involves replacing "it," "they" or "you" with "I." Examples:

1. Change "You are making me angry" to "I am angry." This means the person is owning his own feelings.
2. Change "They say that it will happen in the near future" to "I feel it will happen soon because . . . ." This means the person is owning his own opinion.
3. Change "They—everyone—knows that it is wrong to do that because . . ." to "I feel that it is wrong to do that because . . . ." This means the person is owning his own values.

Talking directly with someone. It can be difficult for some people to talk directly with someone, instead of at or about them. Language is an important part of the contact we make with others; used with directness and precision, it permits us to communicate ourselves. Direct contact with a person can vastly improve communication[17, p. 197].

Problem: John, I don't like the format that JoAnn is using at the curriculum meetings.

Improved: JoAnn, I'm uncomfortable with the way the curriculum meetings are running. I was wondering if the format might be changed?

Processing awareness of bodily sensations. Processing awareness of bodily sensations through immediacy helps a client get in touch with his feelings:

Therapist: How are you feeling right now?
Client: A little upset.
Therapist: What are you sensing with your muscles?
Client: My muscles feel tight. My hands are clenched. My stomach feels like it has been tied in a knot.
Therapist: And this means?
Client: I'm holding myself in. I'm keeping myself from yelling—from screaming. I'm mad—I'm really, really mad. I know that now!

This kind of processing of bodily awareness can be beneficial in dealing with nursing students in helping them to identify their feelings in relation to patient problems and relevant values and issues.

Staying with verbalizing feelings. Staying with verbalizing feelings until they become understood and integrated increases one's awareness and ownership of feelings. The following illustration shows this technique being used in a kindergarten setting[14, p. 77]:

During free choice, John had taken Peter's special STP car. Peter was crying and sobbing, but John wouldn't give it back. I went over and asked what the problem was. John quickly handed Peter his car. Peter was still sobbing. I asked John if he could tell how Peter was feeling.
John: I don't know.
Me: What is he doing?
John: Crying.
Me: Who is crying?
John: Peter is crying.
Me: Do you know how he feels when you take his car?
John: I don't know.
Me: Okay, let me have your shirt. (As I reached out, John stopped me by protecting his shirt. A few tears came into his eyes.) How do you feel if I want to take your shirt?
John: Bad.
Me: Who feels bad?
John: I feel bad.
Me: Do you know how Peter feels now?
John: Yes.

Gestalt philosophy is a specific and ordered way of understanding how we function in the various contexts of our lives. These techniques are ways of implementing the principles and dynamics of this philosophy. They are used according to the particular requirements of each moment during therapy. Sometimes the therapist functions as a technician, using these techniques to point the patient toward new awareness and new risks. Sometimes the encounter (immediacy) between the therapist and the patient is the primary focus of the therapeutic work, so that the therapist's skills focus on that relationship[17, p. 203].

It is important to recognize that in order to be effective, the gestalt therapist, like any therapist, must be in touch with himself, with the patient and with the requirements of the moment. Good therapy demands that the therapist practice what he preaches and provide a good role model. He must be aware of his own self-process and also be aware of his encounter with the patient. In his therapeutic relationships with clients, he must fulfill each of the criteria so aptly identified and described by Rogers: warmth, empathy and congruence[24, pp. xxxi; 9].

Gestalt therapy has been adapted to a variety of settings: schoolrooms, art and modern dance studios, organizations and institutions and natural and planned communities. In psychotherapy it is used in individual, group, couple and family therapy, in workshops, crisis intervention and community mental health settings [17, p. 292]. Many educators believe that development toward self-actualization can be furthered by applying Gestalt philosophy and methodology to education [7].

CONFLUENT EDUCATION

Defined in simple terms, confluent education means putting the whole person—the affective domain (feelings, emotions, attitudes and values) and the cognitive domain (the intellect, the activity of the mind in knowing and thinking)—together into the learning process. Historically in nursing education, however, student needs have been met in an uneven way. Originally, the emphasis was on psychomotor skill development without consideration for cognitive learning. Gradually this changed until recently the emphasis has been on meeting the intellectual needs—what knowledge a nurse must possess in order to provide safe health care. Affective objectives have been set, but the means to meet them has been left relatively undetermined. Confluent education introduces the idea of balance—the integration or flowing together of the affective and cognitive elements in individual and group learning. Putting cognitive and affective elements together through conscious teaching acts is an attempt to make both the educational process and the graduate more humane.

Nursing demands a close association both with people and their problems and with the moral and ethical issues of living. It plays a central role in health counseling and teaching. Its very nature requires effective communication skills on the part of its practitioners. It is our experience that confluent education facilitates the development of these skills through fostering both emotional and intellectual growth of nursing students.

The importance of enhancing both affective and cognitive growth is illustrated in the following situation. A nurse caring for a person who is dying will need cognitive and affective knowledge. The cognitive realm will probably deal with information about the pathological problem affecting the patient's health, level of growth and development, the steps of the grieving process, and so on. The affective realm will include awareness of the nurse's values and feelings about her own mortality and death in general as well as the feelings she has in relation to the patient and his problem. The affective component is especially important, as the nurse will probably have difficulty in dealing effectively with the patient's feelings if she is unaware of her own.

Confluent education can help students to make connections between cognitive and affective elements so that they will be better able to integrate both their thoughts and feelings. It is possible for nurse educators to learn to structure these types of experiences within a nursing curriculum.

According to Yeomans[32, p. 134] confluence is the center of the educational process. He describes confluence as being an experience, not a concept; as something that happens within a person. When it occurs, it has psychological and physiological correlates that can be identified and described. These factors (intellectual and emotional) are joined through the process of confluence into a relationship that leads to the formation of a new whole. The process of confluence includes several steps[32, p. 134]:

1. Interaction: the mutual or reciprocal action or influence of cognitive and affective factors on each other
2. Integration: combining two formerly separate elements (intellect and feelings)
3. Synthesis: joining two or more elements to form a new whole
4. Alignment: there is no conflict between mind and feelings. If alignment is missing, conflict exists causing considerable energy and effort in teaching to be misspent or simply wasted. Another way of looking at this would be to say that if there were alignment between mind and feelings there would be no resistance.

Confluent education is a relatively new type of humanistic education; it provides experiences, some of which use gestalt techniques. Its rapid growth has led to the development of a number of descriptions and terms. As a result, a need arose to clarify them. This need was initially handled by a team from the Development and Research in Confluent Education (DRICE) project supported by the Ford Foundation[27]. The project resulted in a definition of confluent education, a description of some types of education related to it, borderline cases of confluent education, its social context and the practical results that can be anticipated from it[27, pp. 110–113]. The model that resulted from the DRICE project can be useful as a guide in developing confluent nursing education.

Description of Confluent Model

1. Two kinds of learning are fostered simultaneously in confluent education: learning through thinking and learning through doing. Explaining this concept can be difficult because it is complex, controversial and not immediately obvious. For example, in a diad (students in pairs) learning situation, for the first time pairs of students discussed some reading in pharmacology that had been assigned the day before. At the close of the activity, students talked about the experience. They spoke of gaining new awareness of their own strengths and weaknesses in relation to the cognitive subject matter.

—"I need to straighten out the difference between serum and vaccines. I realize that this is important for me to know."
—"Wow, I thought I knew a lot. I now can see I need to reread that chapter."
—"I was able to explain to my partner some definitions that I wasn't too sure of. Now I really know them."
—"I've never done this before. I was uncomfortable, unsure of myself." A response was made to this by another student:
—"I'll bet others felt the same way but were not brave enough to say so." (This exchange highlighted the fact that the uncertain respondent may need help in learning to identify and express her own feelings, or that perhaps an atmosphere of trust among the group members has not yet developed enough for this student to be comfortable in expressing her own feelings.)
—"I didn't expect this kind of experience. It was a little scary."
—"This was fun. I enjoyed doing this. I learned a lot—about me and about pharmacology."

2. There is an open atmosphere so learning may flourish. The structure provides support for both students and teacher to learn. The teacher's responsibility in shaping or setting this kind of climate is to be aware of her own values and the method of reinforcement to student responses.

3. Students and teachers are both urged to express their feelings. Therefore an atmosphere of trust and safety needs to be developed. The teacher needs to establish a role model for students to follow. She also must be nonjudgmental in her responses, to allow for freedom of expression.

4. Experienced-based learning, closely connected to the experiences of the student, is part of confluent education. The learning experience itself leads to inferences and abstractions. For example, a student hearing that she has prepared herself well in one specific area of her education is encouraged to continue to do well in others. Or, several students with clinical experience in caring for patients with similar health problems may be able to draw up a number of broad principles

that would apply to the care of patients with these problems in the future.

5. Feedback is used to clarify and develop all learnings (cognitive and affective). This could be called the observer dimension. The observer (teacher or student) provides feedback in relation to cognitive or affective experience. It is then used to increase the learner's awareness of her strengths and capabilities; it does not judge performance. An approach dealing with the what and how of the situation is essential to the feedback; intrusive "whys" are not part of a confluent approach, which deals with awareness here and now, and makes growth possible. To illustrate: In an experiential activity to teach principles of learning, a diad situation was used. Student A taught Student B something A felt that B should know about controlling hypertension. A was to use appropriate teaching principles. At the end of five minutes, B was to respond to A by sharing what B had learned and to identify the teaching principles that A had used. The instructor provided feedback on whether appropriate attending skills were used[1]. At the close of this experience, students shared with each other the feelings they had during the experience.

—"I can't believe what I learned—things about hypertension, how to teach, how to listen—and I did it all, too!"
—"I learned much more about how I relate to people on a personal basis."
—"I'm excited! A whole lot was going on. I couldn't fall asleep!"
—"I feel better, more confident. If I can teach a classmate, maybe I can teach a patient, too."
—"I heard that I was really doing what I was trying to do and I felt good about that."

6. Developing awareness of self is a legitimate object of learning for both teacher and student. Learning can be directed toward this—what my feelings are, how I relate to people, and so on.

7. Creative and varied thinking is encouraged. The learner has the option to move from personal feelings to cognitive learning, and vice versa.

8. Confluence encourages assimilation and integration of new information, perceptions, and meanings with previous knowledge. As students and teachers share their insights, priorities, and ideas, new perceptions and concepts begin to emerge. The use of group process facilitates this.

9. The transitions between affective and cognitive realms are smooth-flowing, neither extreme nor abrupt. Affect and cognition exist together and their interpenetration is facilitated. A teacher might say, "I feel really good about the feedback I'm about to give you. You had excellent information about the drugs you

were administering. You knew the action, the side effects, pertinent nursing responsibilities and the usual dose of each drug and did not have to refer to your drug cards. Not only that, you also correlated each drug with the patient's specific illness. You have done exceptionally well!" A student, however, might say, "I want to know whether I'm doing well or badly so that I can learn. I want to learn to do things the way they should be done, and I can if you tell me what I'm doing that's right or wrong. I'm really happy that all my work for functional meds was worth it!"

10. The subject matter is directly connected to the personal needs and feelings of the students. In fact, a major factor in the selection of subject materials is the degree to which students can relate to it. For example, a student caring for a patient receiving a blood transfusion will probably develop an interest in knowing about reasons for transfusions, how to administer them and complications that can occur. This material comes to have significant meaning for her as she cares for the patient. She may then transfer some of this significance to other students as she describes her experience to them.

11. Confluent education structures and reinforces the responsibility and accountability of the teacher and students for the integration and growth of the whole person. Self-evaluation of personal growth and evaluations of the performance of the group itself are part of this process.

12. Consideration of resistances to confluent approaches may reveal a need to deal with these before moving on to other learning. For example, a student might complain, "I don't want to try group discussions. You are the most important person to my learning. I want you to lecture. I want to listen to what you have to say." To this, the teacher, beginning to deal with the resistance, replies, "In other words, you want me to be responsible for your learning, and you are feeling uncomfortable with this approach?"

The modes for developing confluent education may create the assumption that it always means a smooth and pleasurable series of cognitive learning events into which affective experience is interjected for excitement. This assumption needs to be corrected where it exists. Confluent education may include situations in which there is a dynamic interplay between affect and cognition that leads to frustration and tension. In appropriate amounts these are viewed as valuable. The interplay can produce a sequence of conflict, persistent confrontation and some degree of resolution or finishing [7, p. 101], which can be quite uncomfortable and difficult for those involved. Dominant members in a group may create this situation, as can disagreements over values, and so forth.

Sometimes, there is concern expressed about whether a teacher is doing teaching or therapy. A teacher is not doing psychotherapy, but should be dealing with the cognitive content of the curriculum and related skills that together represent the learning environment in which she and the students are involved. The affective dimension of the learning situation is the student's response to that environment. This means that the teacher is not a therapist in the sense meant by theories other than Gestalt. A teacher using Gestalt learning principles is not delving into the unconscious motivations of students as would a psychoanalytically oriented therapist. Rather, she is concerned with enhancing the development of human potential—a positive, nonpathological emphasis. This larger purpose is not therapeutic in the narrow sense of the term, although addressing blockages and concerns (resistances to learning) can be remedial in outcome [28, pp. 121-131].

To review the central idea of confluent education, there is no action or learning that does not have both cognitive and affective dimensions. The affective realm may enhance and contribute to cognitive learning or it may cause concerns and resistance. Brown [5, p. 4] divides affective dimensions into loadings and blockages.

Loadings and Blockages

Affective loadings refer to the feeling or emotional aspect of experience and learning: how a person feels about wanting to learn and how he is learning, and what he feels after he has learned. The affective loadings can vary by type and degree depending on the characteristics of the topic—is it interesting and challenging, too hard, too easy, too boring? These affective loadings need to be dealt with in the order in which they occur.

Affective blockages are those underlying psychological concerns of the learner rooted in fundamental (Maslow's hierarchy) human needs [11, p. 50], which, if unmet and ungratified, hinder learning. The basic concerns such as safety, security and self-worth must be fulfilled before the learner can attend to higher needs and goals such as the creative, intellectual or cognitive ones. A teacher focuses on assisting positive affective growth as determined by these hierarchical needs and the response of the learning environment and the student to each other.

It seems important to mention here that it is suspected that gifted teachers for a long time have used the interrelation of affect and cognition to enhance learning [7]. In fact, it is their ability to do so that forms one of the dimensions of their gift. What is new is the concern for program and curriculum development and teacher training in Gestalt therapy that will make this approach possible on a more consistent and widespread basis. Training in Gestalt therapy principles and techniques will be an important aspect of preparation for the teacher in confluent education. This teacher needs to be in touch with herself. This is invaluable. "The good teacher knows himself and knows what is happening NOW. He knows how his students are responding NOW. And he knows what he is doing NOW, how he is doing it, and how he feels as he does it. Experiencing the NOW and taking responsibility for the NOW are essential for successful teaching in confluent education"[5, p. 249]. For some fortunate teachers this is a natural ability, for others it can be a learned skill. Either way, it is essential if one is to foster confluent education, thereby humanizing both nursing education and the graduate nurse.

GROUP PROCESS

The third component of our learning theory is group process—the actual teaching and learning vehicle. The choice of group process as our teaching style is very rational when several factors are considered.

Groups are natural and familiar to us. We are all part of a family group; we live within a neighborhood frequently composed of persons from the same or similar ethnic or socioeconomic group. We participate socially in groups if we are members of a church, a lodge or a social club. Sociologically, these groups share a basic common denominator; they exist because there is mutual interest, communication and dynamic human interaction occurring within them.

Interpersonal relations are vital in our lives. We relate to others constantly, but we relate most openly and significantly when we feel secure, trusting and of value. On a mass level, we are relatively insignificant, defensive and guarded; but in a small group, we feel a sense of well-being and acceptance, thus allowing us to put our defenses down and truly give of ourselves and receive from others. "The group can be considered a small social system which consists of persons influencing and being influenced by one another and drawn together because of similar concerns, goals and values"[15, p. 201]. This type of dynamic interaction is what humanism is all about.

Group Process in Education

Let us look at the use of group process in education and the rationale behind its use. Then we will apply it as a learning tool in a humanistic nursing program.

"Education is a social process. Significant learning occurs through human interaction"[30, p. 2]. Much has been written regarding what should be taught to students and which teaching methods are most effective. As stated earlier, emphasis always has been placed on the cognitive material that must be presented, rather than the form the presentation takes. McLuhan has emphatically stated, "Societies have always been shaped more by the nature of the media by which men communicate than by the content of the communications"[20, p. 8]. Accepting McLuhan's premise, our teaching method then assumes paramount proportions. The "how" of teaching, not the "why," is of major significance. As education occurs through social interactions, we should seek a teaching medium that maximizes these interactions. We believe group process provides us with this medium.

"One of the requirements of a group is that there is interaction and communication among all its members"[21, p. 194]. The traditional classroom in which a teacher faces 25 to 30 students is not a group. Alfred Gorman refers to this type of class as an "aggregate." He goes on to define an aggregate as a collection of people assembled to accomplish a task, but there is an absence of valuable human interaction during the work. Gorman sees aggregate interaction as formal, all members functioning with defenses intact and true feelings carefully held in abeyance. A trusting, sharing relationship does not develop. When the task is completed, the members of the aggregate usually do not really know each other or the teacher[12, p. 3n].

This type of teaching cannot foster interaction among all members without the creation of utter chaos. Tradition dictates that there must be a leader to keep order and direct the class toward task completion. Even teacher-led "group discussions" do not fare well, as usually a few of the more vocal students speak their minds or answer teacher-directed questions, while the vast majority of the class remains quiet, uninvolved and frequently bored. Thus the typical classroom situation does not comprise a group or facilitate group process; its numerical size makes this impossible.

What then does comprise a group? Ideally, a group should consist of six to ten members. These figures may vary as high as 20 or as low as four or five. We have had success in post-clinical conferences with small groups of four students and even frequently engage in one-to-one interaction. In such a small group, each person counts and each has an opportunity to speak, question and share. "Students learn what counts from each other and what society expects from the teacher"[30, p. 3]. If this is so, students must be afforded the opportunity to interact freely and directly with one another.

Humanistic education concerns itself with the development of self-awareness and self-actualization. In order to accomplish this, the student must be allowed to express her thoughts and feelings through her own perceptions. She must feel free to be herself. Further, she must be afforded group feedback in order that she might see herself as others do, and thus evaluate herself. This is of great significance to nursing students, as it gives them an opportunity to evaluate their effects on other people and thereby determine the quality of their interactions.

From our actual experience we have found group process to be a phenomenal learning experience. The reason for this seems to lie in self-involvement. The student is a part of a working group of peers striving toward a common goal, completion of a task assignment that has personal significance. The acquisition of cognitive nursing material pertinent to the current subject is an important goal of the learning process. The facilitation of this goal through group process that fosters affective interaction serves a dual purpose. While working together to acquire the desired knowledge, the group is exposed to an experience in interpersonal relations that allows for true self-expression through relating actual patient care experiences, questioning to clarify gray areas, and genuine reaction and response to the thoughts, ideas, feelings and experiences of other group members. Sharing experiences and ideas provides the opportunity for new concepts and new insights to emerge. One thought or feeling may trigger many new ones among members. The end result of the group experience is more than just a compilation of the input of each member, it is a new whole, for the individual and for the group.

The group acts as an interdependent whole while each part of the whole—i.e., each student—maintains her own independence. For example, a group of five sophomore nursing students was given a pre-clinical conference task of presenting their patient assignments for the day and identifying a major nursing problem they anticipated they would have to cope with in their clinical experience. The group was then to make suggestions on how the anticipated problem might be handled. This is a fairly good method to help a student prepare for a new patient assignment. Following the clinical experience, the group reconvened to discuss briefly what major nursing problems their patients had actually presented.

Student A: Well, when I told you about my patient, Mr. S., with the CVA this morning, I thought my major nursing problem would be dealing with his immobility. It wasn't, he's managing pretty well physically, but his emotional behavior sure threw me.

Student B: How do you mean?

Student A: He'd be talking fine, even laughing then suddenly he'd start crying for no reason. I really felt uncomfortable. I didn't know what to do.

Student B: Hmm, you don't know whether to stay or run! (Laughter among the group—recognition of a common problem.)

Student C: I had a CVA patient last semester like that. Apparently, the mood swings are a part of the disease process. I remember reading about it in our book.

Student A: Really! I kept trying to find a concrete reason for each crying episode. It was really getting to me. I don't feel so bad now.

Student D (to the entire group): But what do you do when a patient starts to cry?

A lively conversation ensued, with each student relating appropriate past clinical experiences with crying patients and how they handled or mishandled the situations. Additional cognitive knowledge emerged and personal feelings regarding a common problem were expressed. From these revelations, a sharing process occurred to help each member find a way to cope with the problem.

The student who expressed concern over the problem felt secure enough to state her feelings of inadequacy to the group. Other members acknowledged that they also had these feelings. A self-awareness of their feelings in the given situation helped clarify how their own emotions were impeding their nursing care. The group as a whole then discussed methods for dealing with their feelings and subsequently with patients' feelings.

The group continued their conversation after post-clinical conference had concluded, and as they headed out of the hospital, they were still carrying on a lively discussion.

Through a basic task assignment, new information was learned, and a learning need of importance to the group members emerged. The members related strongly to the need, shared their experiences, applied mental health principles in their discussion and came up with some suggestions for alternative ways to handle the situation. Self-awareness, growth and confluence were fostered by way of the group process.

Objectives of Group Process

Carl Rogers states that the intensive group experience is one of the most effective means available to facilitate learning, growth and positive change in the student [25, p. 304]. As these are our major humanistic teaching goals, it behooves us to clarify how group process helps accomplish them. Our basic objectives for the use of group process are:

1. To impart cognitive information pertinent and relevant to the practice of nursing.
2. To foster an environment conducive to dynamic human interaction.
3. To encourage integration of theoretical and experiential learning through participation.
4. To facilitate the development of a self-actualized person by way of a humanistic teaching method that allows each student to recognize and strive toward full potential.

Each student learns to listen to others and experiences being listened to by others; this fosters awareness of others' feelings and an increased insight into one's own. As commonalities of experience emerge, the student feels freer to express herself, and thus gains in self-awareness. As others in the group experience this freedom of expression and share their feelings, each student develops a greater awareness of the feelings of others.

Interaction among the group members allows for acceptance and respect for others and self to develop. This type of humanistic behavior learned and experienced in group process can allow for behavior changes that the student will carry over into her relationships with patients, staff and all persons with whom she comes in contact.

The method is affective, the content is cognitive, but the two mesh through the process of human dynamics, and with that mesh, confluence is achieved.

The learning has been personalized by the group and by each member within it. The freedom group process provides allows the student to be herself, non-defensive and open to change. It allows her to become a more self-actualizing person— the goal of humanistic education.

These, of course, are the ideal goals of group process and not accomplished without a conducive environment, a facilitative teacher and an understanding of group members' responsibilities. These issues will be discussed in depth in Chapter 4.

REFERENCES

1. Anthony, W., and Carkhuff, R. *The Art of Health Care: A Handbook of Psychological First Aid Skills.* Amherst, Mass.: Human Resources Development Press, 1976.
2. Aspy, D. *Toward a Technology for Humanizing Education.* Champaign, Ill.: Research Press, 1972.
3. Beisser, A. Paradoxical Theory. In J. Fagan and I. Shephard (Eds.), *Gestalt Therapy Now.* New York: Harper and Row, 1970.
4. Borton, T. *Reach, Touch, Teach.* New York: McGraw-Hill, 1970.
5. Brown, G. Human Is as Confluent Does. In G. I. Brown, T. Yeomans and L. Grizzard (Eds.) *The Live Classroom.* New York: Viking, 1975.
6. Brown, G. *Human Teaching for Human Learning.* New York: Viking, 1971.
7. Brown, G.; Yeomans, T.; and Grizzard, L. (Eds.). *The Live Classroom.* New York: Viking, 1975.
8. Egan, G. *The Skilled Helper.* Monterey, Calif.: Brooks/Cole, 1975.
9. Evans, R. *Carl Rogers, The Man and His Ideas.* New York: Dutton, 1975.
10. Fagan, J., and Shepherd, I. *Gestalt Therapy Now.* New York: Harper and Row, 1970.
11. Goble, F. *The Third Force.* New York: Grossman, 1970.
12. Gorman, A. *Teachers and Learners: The Interactive Process.* Boston: Allyn and Bacon, 1969.
13. Greenberg, H. *Teaching with Feeling.* New York: Macmillan, 1969.
14. Grizzard, V. Gestalt and the Substitute Teacher. In G. I. Brown; T. Yeomans; and L. Grizzard (Eds.); *The Live Classroom.* New York: Viking, 1975.
15. Heidgerkin, L. *Teaching and Learning in Schools of Nursing: Principles and Methods.* Philadelphia: Lippincott, 1965.
16. James, M., and Jongeward, D. *Born to Win.* Reading, Mass.: Addison-Wesley, 1971.
17. Latner, J. *The Gestalt Therapy Book.* New York: Julian Press, 1973.
18. Mann, J. *Learning to Be.* New York: Free Press, 1972.
19. McCarthy, D. Gestalt as Learning Theory. In G. I. Brown; T. Yeomans; and L. Grizzard (Eds.), *The Live Classroom.* New York: Viking, 1975.
20. McLuhan, M., and Fiore, Q. *The Medium Is the Massage.* New York: Random House, 1967.
21. Patterson, C. *Humanistic Education.* Englewood Cliffs, N.J.: Prentice-Hall, 1973.
22. Perls, F. *Gestalt Therapy Verbatim.* Lafayette, Calif.: Real People Press, 1969.
23. Perls, F. Four Lectures In J. Fagen and I. Shepherd (Eds.), *Gestalt Therapy Now.* New York: Harper and Row, 1970.
24. Perls, F.; Hefferline, R.; and Goodman, P. *Gestalt Therapy.* New York: Julian Press, 1951.
25. Rogers, C. *Freedom to Learn.* Columbus, Ohio: Charles E. Merrill, 1969.
26. Rogers, C., and Stevens, B. *Person to Person: The Problem of Being Human. A New Trend in Psychology.* Lafayette, Calif.: Real People Press, 1967.
27. Shapiro, S. Developing Models by Unpacking Confluent Education. In G. I. Brown; T. Yeomans; and L. Grizzard (Eds.), *The Live Classroom.* New York: Viking, 1975.
28. Shiflett, J. Beyond Vibration Teaching: Research and Curriculum Development in Confluent Education. In G. I. Brown; T. Yeomans; and L. Grizzard (Eds.), *The Live Classroom.* New York: Viking, 1975.
29. Simkin, J. An Introduction to Gestalt Therapy. In G. I. Brown; T. Yeomans; and L. Grizzard (Eds.), *The Live Classroom.* New York: Viking, 1975.
30. Stanford, G., and Roark, A. *Human Interaction in Education.* Boston: Allyn and Bacon, 1974. Available from Dr. Gene Stanford, Children's Hospital, 219 Bryant Street, Buffalo, NY 14222.
31. Wilson, J. *Thinking with Concepts.* Cambridge, England: Cambridge University Press, 1963.
32. Yeomans, T. Search for a Working Model: Gestalt, Psychosynthesis, and Confluent Education. In G. I. Brown; T. Yeomans; and L. Grizzard (Eds.) *The Live Classroom.* New York: Viking, 1975.

CHAPTER 4

The Method of Group Process

Group process has made it possible for us to implement confluent nursing education. Personal experience leaves no doubt in our minds that this method succeeds in enhancing effective and dynamic communication between teachers and students and among students. We have found the result to be an intellectual and personal growth for all concerned.

We feel that extensive interdependence exists between effective communication and group process development. As effective communication is developed, the dynamics of group process are enhanced; as the dynamics of group development are fostered, communication is improved. We have discovered that encouraging the simultaneous development of both of these essential, separate yet interdependent elements is the key to fostering confluent nursing education.

Let us take a look at a classroom. Although there may be 20 to 30 students, they may not constitute a group; effective communication may or may not be present. Those classes that do become productive working groups share certain characteristics in common[22, p. 26] : the members understand and accept each other, each person takes responsibility for her own learning and actions, members cooperate and are helpful to each other, methods for making decisions have been established, communication is open, and members are able to confront problems openly and settle their conflicts constructively. Unfortunately, groups like this do not magically occur. They need to be carefully nurtured.

It is possible to assess the degree to which a class of students manifests the properties of a group and to place it somewhere on a continuum between nongroup and group. The extent to which a class of students moves along the continuum toward becoming a productive working group depends on both teacher and students. Every person has a responsible role to play in enhancing both effective communication and the development of the class toward becoming a group. In this chapter, we will review the use of effective communication and group dynamics essential to fostering group process in nursing education.

COMMUNICATION

Good communication can diminish disruptive group behavior and encourage greater participation and sharing on the part of each member. According to Schmuck and Schmuck[20] effective communication can foster the type of classroom environment that enhances a student's feelings of being accepted and belonging, of having some power in the sense of being able to influence the ideas and learnings of teacher and classmates, and of feeling competent and successful from experiencing achievement. A student who is able to have these basic needs fulfilled can direct her energy toward other goals of intellectual and personal growth. Concurrent with working toward her other goals, however, she must be responsible for helping to maintain the kind of environment that will fulfill the basic needs for belonging, control and achievement. As a group develops and the students grow toward greater interdependence, the reality of Glasser's[12] concept of individual responsibility, "the ability to fulfill one's needs and to do so in a way that does not deprive others of the ability to fulfill their need," becomes even more crucial. Members grow to trust and rely on each other. They become more willing to risk and share themselves.

Fostering effective communication is the responsibility of the teacher as well as the student. In order for us as teachers to accept and meet this responsibility more fully than we had done in our previous teaching, we found it necessary to increase our own growth and development in communication. This meant achieving a greater personal knowledge of and more conscious awareness of effective and ineffective communication, as well as cultivating improved basic and advanced communication skills. We have discovered this to be an ever-deepening, perpetual learning process.

Eventually as our own foundation in communication became secure, using a counseling model we began to teach basic communication skills of accurate understanding (empathy) to students in our clinical groups to enhance effective communication and to encourage group process development. While some of these skills had been introduced in earlier courses that presented basic principles of interviewing techniques and psychiatric nursing, the level of skill development varied greatly from student to student. Most needed a review and further encouragement and reinforcement to transfer them into everyday use.

The experience that we have integrated into our clinical conferences is patterned after Carkhuff's counseling model[6] and can be classified as human relations training or training in the helping process. The skills are designed to assist students in using certain core conditions of effective communication. These core conditions include empathy, warmth, respect, genuineness, self-disclosure, concreteness, confrontation, and immediacy. According to Gazda[10, p. 13] this selection of conditions has been identified and supported with impressive research as being fundamental to effective communication. Individuals who are functioning at high levels of interpersonal effectiveness are able to use these conditions to help people move through various phases of the decision–making process. Cark-huff[1] identifies the phases of this process as exploration, understanding, and action.

Our clinical format provides experiential learning of communication skills that convey these conditions. The students both listen and are listened to. The skill to be practiced is defined in a task set by the instructor, but the individual student selects the agenda to share with a fellow group member or members, according to what is important to her. Students practice the selected communication skill while they are listening and responding to each other. For example, they may share with each other something important that they learned, their reactions to what has happened to them during their clinical experience, their feelings concerning certain ethical issues and differences in values or a personal problem they feel comfortable in discussing. Through the medium of interpersonal relations, the students experience the message — the importance of using effective communication skills[16].

As these skills are developed and practiced in conference, they can be transferred into use with patients and their families, peers, teachers, families and friends. As individuals become more proficient, they have a tendency to move from a situation of mechanical and awkward usage of them to one of owning or living them automatically. They can become a way of life.

Modes of Nonverbal Communication

As an introduction, we frequently begin with activities in the vital area of nonverbal communication. Nonverbal communication is broadly defined by Gazda [10, p. 88] as "any human behavior that is directly perceived by another person and that is informative about the sender." A few examples for illustration might be: facial expression, the position a person takes in a room, eye contact, hand gestures, posture, style of dress, loudness of voice, arrangement of furniture, touching. Often nonverbal communication conveys more of the meaning behind what a person is saying than do the words he is using.

We introduce several aspects of this modality to our clinical groups: (1) observation and identification of nonverbal behavior in group members and the reactions of other members to it; (2) interpretation of the meaning of nonverbal behavior in relation to a person's concerns, feelings, self-concept and energy level; and (3) attending skills—nonverbal communication of the helper.* Each of these areas will be discussed separately.

---

*Note on terminology:

Person who is seeking help: In medical and nursing circles, the person coming for help has always been called the patient. This has been true for patients with physical as well as emotional problems. In counseling, Rogers introduced the word client and used it extensively[8]. This helped

Observation and Identification. Students are helped to experience and to identify types of nonverbal behavior in other group members and to describe their own reactions to it. To accomplish this, activities are developed in which students are assigned specific nonverbal roles to play. For illustration, in a situation with three students (triad), Student A is assigned to be the speaker (helpee) and to talk about something of significance to her. Student B is assigned to be the listener (helper) and to display a particular type of nonverbal behavior while she is listening to A. Student C is assigned the role of observer. She is to give feedback to A and B about their behavior, and her reactions to it.

Sample activity While A is talking, B may be asked to drum her fingers, shift in her seat, look at her watch, fold her arms across her chest, look out the window. At the end of three to five minutes, A is asked to stop talking about her chosen topic and to describe to B how she felt about B's behavior. Student A may describe feelings of rejection or hurt when Student B drummed her fingers or checked her watch. Student C, as observer, describes the behavior that she observed occurring in A and B throughout their entire exchange, and her reactions to what was happening. Remaining in their groups of three, students are then asked to share with each other what they learned about themselves during this experience. Nonverbal assignments are changed and rotated until every student has had an opportunity to experience each role.

Results On a Gestalt level, this experience provides a student with practice being more in touch with her feelings in the here and now and provides opportunity for her to express them. On a different level, it emphasizes the meaning and effect nonverbal behavior can have on people. All of this is accomplished through experiential learning with the whole student—mind, body and feelings—involved.

Interpretation

A second aspect of nonverbal communication has to do with learning to observe carefully the behavior of another person, and to interpret the meaning that it has in relation to that person's concerns, feelings, self-concept and energy level. This

counseling move away from the medical model. The word helpee is also currently being used in order to denote the "person coming for help." Throughout the remaining chapters, we use a variety of these terms to identify the person seeking help. In addition, the word *speaker* or *talker* is also used to mean the person playing the role of the helpee in the experiential learning activities that we describe.

Person (nurse) who is doing the helping: The person who supplies the help or counseling is identified as the nurse, helper, counselor, listener, or responder.

skill is relatively easy for nursing students to master, because they are already familiar with observing patients carefully for changes in their clinical signs and symptoms that provide information about their physical condition. Some caution needs to be introduced, however, as various nonverbal behaviors can have different meanings to different people: i.e., arms crossed might mean "I'm cold," "I'm bored," "It's a comfortable position," "I'm nervous."

One area of observation on which students are encouraged to focus attention is the helpee's energy level[6]. When a person's energy level is low, he functions poorly. If it is high, he is more apt to function effectively. Students are familiar with the fact that low energy levels are apt to exist in people because of illness, and that this makes it difficult for people to meet even the simplest demands of everyday life. They learn also that some of the low energy levels may be caused by conflicts within a person. Because conflicts are draining his energy, a person may be fatigued, slow to respond and often act inappropriately to a situation. He may perceive his everday life as overwhelming; everything is a burden. Students learn to observe a person's posture, body build, grooming and nonverbal behavior to provide clues about his energy level. Even a person's voice, the loudness or softness, pitch, tone and spacing of words, help in this assessment.

In addition to assessing energy level, students learn to discern whether or not a person is congruent. Are there discrepancies or inconsistencies in his behavior? Does he say he is happy yet have a sad facial expression? How in touch with his feelings, values and inner self is he? All of these observations bring us closer to understanding another person's world a little better.

An activity for learning these concepts may be one that involves small groups of four or five students. Student volunteers are used to model various nonverbal behaviors that convey feelings. Group members are asked to list individually as many meanings for a particular nonverbal behavior as they can, and pool them into one list from each group. These lists are compared and discussed in the whole conference group. Students are asked to share their reactions and what they learned about themselves from this activity.

Attending Skills. The third aspect of nonverbal communication has to do with the behavior of the person who is doing the helping. This involves the concept of attending skills which in Carkhuff's counseling model are the very foundation of the helping process[6]. In general, attending can be defined as being attentive to the person with whom you are having a conversation. The physical attention that is provided by a helper listening to a person talk can communicate interest, respect, concern and involvement.

In conference, students practice attending to each other in diad, triad and small group situations. Egan's SOLER description of attending skills[9] is used as a norm for them to use when giving feedback to each other about their attending behavior.

The SOLER model[9, p. 114] identifies five basic things that a person can do with his body to convey that he is interested and involved with the individual to whom he is listening:

S: Face the person *squarely,* shoulder to shoulder. In a group setting one can turn in some way toward the person speaking.
O: Maintain an *open posture,* especially open arms, not crossed, to indicate that one is open to that other person, to what he or she wants to say.
L: *Lean* slightly forward toward the other person. Again, this is another sign of caring, being involved, being available.
E: Maintain good *eye contact.* Sometimes there is concern that direct eye contact may be uncomfortable, may be seen as staring the other person down. Yet people really involved with each other have almost constant eye contact.
R: Be *relaxed* or at ease. If one is tense and rigid, this is often what is communicated to the person with whom you are involved in conversation.

While a student is beginning her practice of attending skills, she is in a triad setting and listening to a student share what was important to her about her clinical experience that day. A third person observes and eventually gives feedback to the listening student about her attending behavior. At the end of the exercise an opportunity is provided for the students to share with each other their reactions to this experience and what they learned about themselves.

Attending skills are the foundation of the communication process. Lack of them communicates, "You're not listening to me!" Such inattention is annoying because it seems to reflect lack of respect for the helpee by the helper. Respect has been identified as one of the fundamental elements that is vital to effective communication. According to Egan[9, p. 122], good attending behavior, including the ability to identify feelings and the experiences and behaviors that underlie them, provides the basis for understanding or empathy, which means appreciating someones else's world, seeing things from another person's point of view.

The next step in communication, as in counseling, is for the listener to try to communicate to the person talking some of her understanding about the helpee's feelings, appearance, behavior, energy level, consistencies and inconsistencies. This type of communication, however, needs to be done tentatively. It also requires that a foundation of trust be built up between the two people involved.

This brings us to the next section of communication, which deals with verbal responding skills that can convey empathy. For a person to be effective, whether communicating in everyday relationships or in the helping process, it is essential that she be able to convey empathy.

Levels of Verbal Responses in Communication

It is generally accepted that the majority of human behaviors are learned through the interactions of people with their environment. When interaction occurs in the area of interpersonal relationships, it greatly influences development of communication skills. Through these relationships people learn who they are, what they are and how to respond to each other. Their responses form the basis for communication. Some are helpful, others are harmful; some are effective, others are ineffective.

In his counseling model, Carkhuff[6] identifies five levels of verbal responding that constitute varying degrees of effectiveness in interpersonal communication:

Level 1: Very ineffective, not helpful at all as the response is *totally unrelated* and irrelevant to the speaker's expression.

Level 2: Ineffective, as it does *not* respond to the *feelings* expressed by the speaker although it may be related to the content of what was said.

Level 3: Minimally effective to effective, because it identifies and reflects the speaker's *feeling* and gives a paraphrase of the *content* of what he said. It is primary level *empathy* response: content plus feelings equals meaning. It conveys understanding.

Level 4: Very effective because it includes the content and feelings of the speaker, and it responds to where the speaker is and where he wants to be. It is a *personalizing* response that helps the speaker accept responsibility for himself.

Level 5: Extremely effective because it goes beyond Level 4 to provide not only a response with accurate content and feelings, related to where the speaker is and where he wants to be, but also includes steps for *action* (how to get from where the helpee is to where he wants to be). It is an *initiating* response. It suggests action.

To illustrate the five levels, we have included a description of a situation that involved a student during a recent clinical experience. Following the episode, examples of each of the levels of responding are included. She might have selected any one of them to use in making her response. We would hope that she learned in our clinical sessions to make an empathic response. Can you select which one that would be?

Situation. On the second day the student is caring for the patient, the patient's wife says, "I'm wondering what to do. You know he made this decision by himself to have this treatment and look what's happened to him. He's so sick! And there's no one who can answer my questions. Why did this happen? What's going on? I can't find anyone to talk to. I really don't want all these people coming in and bothering him any more. It's just too hard on him. Look how sick he is now."

Response Options.

A. In other words, you're afraid and upset with yourself, too, because you're not sure how to go about making a big decision and it's important for you to make a good one—a right one for your husband's well-being. A first step might be for us to sit down and talk over some of the things that are bothering you and perhaps I can answer your questions, too.

B. You're saying you don't know what to do and nobody is here to help you find the answers.

C. You seem to feel pretty upset and mixed up because your husband became ill after his treatment, and worst of all, no one is helping you sort out what's happening.

D. It's the team approach, and it's really pretty good, once you get use to dealing with it and the different people.

E. It seems that you're upset with yourself and feeling helpless because you want to do what's best for your husband in this situation; but you're not sure just how to weigh things out and you want to do this and make a right decision, one that will help your husband.

The responses made here match up with Carkhuff's descriptive model in the following way:

A is a Level 5 response because it includes the speaker's content and reflects her feelings. It conveys understanding of where the person is and where he wants to go and includes steps for action to get there.

B is a Level 2 response because it refers to the content only of what the speaker has said.

C is a Level 3 response because it includes content and reflects feelings. It conveys empathy.

D is a Level 1 response because it is unrelated to what the speaker is actually saying.

E is a Level 4 response because it includes content plus feelings, as well as a statement about where the helpee is now in relation to where she wants to be.

Response Levels 1 and 2 lead to ineffective communication. Response Levels 3 through 5 constitute effective communication and what Carkhuff[6] describes as being the helping process. When these levels are used appropriately in responding, a helper is able to facilitate the movement of a helpee through the various stages of the learning or decision-making process. A nurse can use the helping process to assist a patient in exploring his situation, understanding it, making decisions and acting upon them. In the sample situation, the student was able to initiate such communication with the patient's wife.

The learning or decision-making process is common to each of us. Periodically, people may need varying degrees of assistance in order to make a decision and affect some changes in their lives. It is important for a person to explore each stage of the process fully as he proceeds, because the process itself is developmental, with each stage building on the one preceding it.

Carkhuff[6] provides a developmental map of the learning or decision-making process. *Self-exploration* is the first phase, exploring where we are in relation to our world and the people in it and examining our values. *Understanding* is the second phase, understanding where we are in relation to where we want to be, accepting responsibility for ourselves and be where we are at any given moment. *Action* is the third phase, taking actual steps to move from where we are to where we want to be. Figure 4–1 shows how the response Levels 3, 4 and 5 of the *helping process* correspond to the phases of the *learning process* [6].

Our aim is to provide students with an overview of the total communication process and with practice in making Level 3 responses. Responding to each other on this level enables the students to convey empathy. The next step is for them to transfer this level of responding into their communication with patients. When they are able to communicate accurate understanding to other people, they can participate more effectively not only in their clinical group, but ultimately in all their relationships.

Frequently, some students who are naturally empathic move beyond making a primary empathy response. Others may have extreme difficulty reaching the point at which they can make even a minimal Level 3 response. Student comments from year to year substantiate the need for this kind of experience in communicating. Frequently, we listen to statements similar to the following:

"I want to help my patients. I want to say something, but I don't know what to say. I work so hard on concentrating on what I should say that would make a good 'process recording' response that I miss what the patient is really saying."

"I can't find the right words. I don't want to say something that might hurt."

"I get scared—what will I say?"

"How will I answer a patient who asks me a difficult question like, 'Do I have cancer?'"

"Isn't it okay to tell a patient there's always hope? Doesn't everyone always, deep down, believe there is hope?"

Figure 4-1. Correspondence of the helping process to the learning process

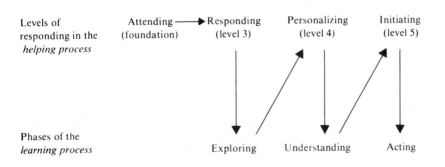

"She's so lonely, but I don't know how to talk with her. She might cry."

"I feel so strongly negative about what this patient is doing and yet I don't want her to do what I want, I want her to do what is best for her, and I don't know how to make this happen."

We have found that introducing students to making and experiencing Level 3 empathic responses in a structured group setting has been extremely helpful in assisting them to overcome their deficiencies and their anxieties about communicating therapeutically. Confidence in their ability to communicate with empathy grows as they experience struggling with, and finally making, a Level 3 response. Whether it is or is not a Level 3 statement is usually made clear by responses from the student helpee and from an objective student observer. The criterion for assessing the quality of the response is Carkhuff's description of a Level 3 response: content plus feelings equals meaning. Students share their reactions to the responses and to the total learning experience.

Skills of Communication

The skills of communication that we assist the students to practice during conference are the basic skills of attending and responding at Level 3. Other more advanced skills in communicating are demonstrated and used as the need arises during the semester. Confrontation, immediacy, concreteness versus vagueness and self-disclosure are examples of these more advanced skills. As the students have already developed a basic background in responding with understanding to each other, a firm foundation exists for introducing the more advanced skills whenever a situation arises that demands their use. Often conflicts over individual responsibility, domineering autocractic leadership of one student, lack of participation by some members or failure to fulfill helpful group roles may lead to the need for intervening with confrontation and immediacy.

There are three essential parts to any level of interpersonal communication skill. These are awareness of perception, communication know-how and assertiveness[9]. Nursing students are quick in being able to identify these critical ingredients. Their ability to implement the skills improves with practice.

Awareness of Perception. There is an awareness of perception part to every communication skill. "Learning how to pay closer attention to yourself, to others, and to the situation in which you find yourself relating to others, is necessary if you're going to develop the kind of awareness that is the foundation of interpersonal skills"[9, p. 39].

In relation to self-awareness and perception, many nursing students are in touch with themselves and are able to identify and share their own feelings. Others need assistance with this.

Example 1 Instructor: You seemed angry after conference this morning—perhaps because you received so little support or help this morning.

Student A: Oh, yes! I was angry, but I was also feeling very lonely and isolated. No one seemed to care enough to help me out. I'm mostly angry at myself, though, because I didn't do anything about what was happening.

Example 2: Setting: a learning situation in which students are asked to share their reactions to an experience with each other.

Student B: This is silly. I don't have any feelings one way or the other. I don't see the purpose of this.

For Student B, self-disclosure of any kind seems to pose a threat. It is hoped that through her observations and her experience interacting with peers such as Student A, who are willing to share their feelings about a particular situation, she will develop an awareness of her difficulty in this area. It is also possible, however, that her resistance may be great enough to interfere with her gaining this awareness and participating as an effective group member.

Most nursing students usually can recognize the feelings that another is displaying with nonverbal behavior because they are familiar with making observations of patients. It is knowing how to communicate this information to the person involved that presents some difficulty. Conference time provides for practice in this area.

Communication Know-how. "Your awareness or perception of yourself or another person can only be put to use if you know how to communicate this awareness to others" [9, p. 39]. Being able to convey your perceptions to someone clearly, concisely and in a non-threatening or non-challenging manner is important. While students are practicing their communication skills, their feedback to each other frequently highlights these points.

Anne (as observer): Sarah, you sounded to me like you were diagnosing Mary and telling her what her feelings really were. You were coming across pretty strong.

Mary: Well, I felt myself feeling defensive and sort of angry.

Sarah: I hear you both saying that I need to be softer, more tentative in my approach, not accusing in the way I tell someone my perceptions.

To summarize, good perceptions must go hand in hand with good communication know-how for skillful communication to occur.

Assertiveness. Assertive behavior refers to the student actually putting the communication skills into use. She does so in a way that respects her own rights and the rights of other people. "High-quality awareness and excellent communication know-how are meaningless unless you have the courage to use them" [9, p. 39].

During a discussion about pharmacology, a student offered a correct answer to a group quiz question. The rest of the group members were unfamiliar with the information the student was providing and tended to ignore her. She presented the information several times, but no one acknowledged it. Consequently, the group got the quiz question wrong.

Student A: Well, that's me, I knew I had read that information somewhere. I'm just not assertive enough, that's all. I'll have to remember this for next time.

Student B: Yes but I didn't pay as much attention to you as I should have. None of us did.

Students were recognizing problems with assertiveness and listening, as well as setting some goals for personal growth.

Description of Communication Skills

Attending. Attending means being actively present to another person. Body language carries the message, 'I'm interested in you. I'm available to you right now. I respect you." As a norm for their attending skills, students use Egan's [9] SOLER (see page 64).

Responding with Understanding. Being able to communicate understanding to another person is not the whole of the interpersonal communication process, but it is basic to building trust and forming a foundation for the use of more advanced communication skills when they are needed. According to Carkhuff [6], content plus feelings will convey an accurate level of understanding. This response has two vital components: (1) the surface feelings of the helpee, perceived by the helper, and (2) the content that includes the life experiences and behaviors of the helpee that give rise to his feelings. Students learn this response in three steps. First, they practice responding by paraphrasing the content of what they heard the helpee say. Second, they respond only by reflecting the feelings they perceived. Third, they combine the two by reflecting the feelings and paraphrasing the content in one statement. Consider the following illustration:

Student A: I never seem to be able to study enough to get ahead, and I'm feeling very tired, really exhausted. I can't wait to finish all this. It's just too much: children, home, working, going to school. I need a vacation.

Response step 1: Paraphrasing content

Student B: In other words, the pressure from all these demands on you is mounting up and becoming overwhelming.

Response step 2: Reflecting feelings

Student C: I sense you're feeling discouraged and down.

Response step 3: Reflecting feelings and paraphrasing content

Student D: I sense you're feeling discouraged and down because there is no relief from this mounting responsibility and pressure.

Each of these steps is introduced individually, and the students practice them in role-playing triad situations.

Step 1: Paraphrasing content. Content includes the various experiences and behaviors that give rise to a person's feelings. It is necessary to refer to content in order to convey understanding of the person's situation as he sees it. The following formula is suggested for use by the students until they have sufficient mastery of the skill of responding with feelings and content. Then they may use language that is more natural to them and therefore less artificial sounding.

Formula: "In other words, you are saying . . . [paraphrase the content] ."

Students take turns in being the helpee, the helper and observer in a triad setting. The helpee shares a problem or describes her learning experience for one to two minutes. The helper in 15 to 30 seconds responds to the helpee using the formula, "In other words, you are saying. . . ." The observer gives feedback to the helper about her use of the formula, her paraphrasing accuracy and her attending skills. She shares her own reactions to the response. The helpee also shares her reactions to the response. All students discuss their reactions to the experience.

Step 2: Reflecting feelings. Feelings are the emotions that a person is experiencing. Once you have identified the feelings another person is experiencing, the next step is to express understanding of them to the other person. The following formula is suggested for use while students are learning this skill.

Formula: "I sense you feel . . . [feeling word or phrase] ."

Students take turns in being the helpee, the helper and the observer in a triad setting. The helpee shares a personal problem or describes her learning experience for one to two minutes. The helper in 15 to 30 second responds to the helpee using the formula, "I sense you feel. . . ." The exercise continues as in step 1.

Step 3: Responding with content and feelings. Making a combined interchangeable response communicates initial basic understanding of what the helpee is feeling and the experiences behind these feelings. It is a Level 3 "content plus feelings equals meaning" response. Use of this combined response, for example, allows a student to convey to her patient that she understands his world from his frame of reference. The following formula is suggested for use until mastery of the skill is sufficient to allow the student to convey the same message, but in a more natural-sounding manner:

Formula: "I sense you feel . . . [feeling word or phrase] because . . . [paraphrase of content] ."

Students take turns in being the helpee, the helper and the observer in a triad setting. The exercise proceeds as in the previous two steps, except that the helper uses the formula, "I sense you feel . . . because. . . ."

Student responses to the learning of these skills have been very positive. It tends to provide them with a concrete way of dealing with the otherwise abstract concept of empathy. Not only do they practice the skill, but they also experience what it feels like to be on the receiving end, what it is like to experience empathy. Some of their reactions to learning the skills are as follows:

—"This is hard, but I like it. There are no gimmicks. I just concentrate on what the patient is saying."
—"I have to listen hard. I don't worry quite as much about what I'm going to say."
—"This is better than asking questions. I don't like to be asked questions. People seem to keep right on talking if I use this approach."
—"The words make me sound automatic and stiff. Will I be that way after I use them awhile?"
—"I know better what to say now. It sort of comes from the patient, not from me!"

As the semester progresses, and students have mastered the basic empathy response, other more advanced skills are introduced when the occasion arises.

Concrete Response. At various times, a summary of the issues a helper has raised can be used effectively. It can add direction and coherence to a helpee's self-exploration that has been confused and rambling.

Student: There seem to be several areas that are concerning you now: your relationship with your husband, facing your children and friends, coping with your own acceptance of the changes in you. Perhaps you're worried that people's reactions, your own and others, are going to bring about hurtful changes in your life.

Patient: Yes, that sort of sums it all up. I'm scared to death that I'm going to lose everything and that I can't control the outcome. Oh, I want desperately to be the same me—the same person I was before.

The skill of concreteness includes three elements: specific experiences, specific behaviors and specific feelings and emotions. This example included two of these aspects—experiences and emotions. Any one of these three elements can be used in combination with another and sometimes separately. The important idea is to be specific and not abstract or vague. Concreteness helps to avoid misunderstandings and game playing.

Vague Response. A vague response by a helper when the helpee has been dealing with a concrete situation allows the helpee to select whatever aspect of the situation she wishes to discuss. It allows her control and direction over the discussion.

A patient was told the preceding day that she had cancer. The doctor telling her this said at that time that he had developed a plan for her to receive chemotherapy treatment, the purpose of which was to take care of any of the cancer cells that might have been left behind by the surgery. The patient was to receive the chemotherapy on five consecutive days out of every month. The doctor then reviewed the side effects of the therapy and asked the patient if she had any questions. When she had none, he left.

Student (next morning): I'm concerned about you and about your reactions to the news you received from Dr. R yesterday.
Patient: Well, I'm really worried about how I'm going to manage getting the chemotherapy five days each month and still go to my job in the city. (The patient commuted by train to New York City from a suburb 50 miles away.)

This response allowed the patient to direct the discussion to the area that was of most concern to her at the moment. The student was surprised, as she expected the patient to talk about her feelings in relation to having cancer. This approach helped the student to deal with the patient's needs as the patient perceived them differently from the student.

Self-Disclosure. Self-disclosure involves sharing something about one's own personal life. The value of doing this in a counseling situation is in question[8, p. 155]. Egan[8] describes two contradictory sets of evidence: one set urges helper self-disclosure, while the other cautions against it. On the one hand, Weigel and associates have evidence suggesting that the helper's self-disclosure can frighten the helpee or make the helper seem less effective[8]. On the other hand, Jourard's approach is that by modeling self-disclosure, the helper can help the client learn how to disclose himself more effectively[8].

From our experience, we feel that students at this stage in their development of counseling and communication are not ready to use this skill in therapeutic communication with their patients. We do, however, accept Jourard's idea that self-disclosure is an essential part of the process of self-actualization. We encourage a student to recognize and be in touch with her feelings related to her learning during conference and clinical experience caring for patients. She is encouraged to share these feelings with other group members. In addition, when she is talking about a problem during a discussion or triad activity, the helper's response will assist her to be in touch with her feelings at that time, a phenomenon Rogers describes as congruence[18].

Confrontation. This is a response that "invites a person to examine his or her interpersonal style—emotions, experiences, and behaviors—and its consequences (for instance, how it affects others) more carefully"[9, p. 211]. Through confrontation, it is possible to challenge the discrepancies, distortions, games and unwillingness to understand the unproductive behaviors that plague our interpersonal lives. In order for confrontation to promote growth, it must be done in a positive, caring and responsible way.

There are five different kinds of confrontation[9, pp. 212-218]: information, experiential, strength, weakness and encouragement to action.

Information confrontation: In information confrontation, the helper supplies the helpee with some information that he needs in order to involve himself more effectively with others.

> Student A: You are always prepared, but you rarely talk in the group. I wish you would share more. I could learn a lot from you.
> Student B: I would like to talk more, but I don't have a chance because you do most of the talking.
> Student A: I do? I didn't realize that.
> Student B: Well, you do. I hardly have a chance to say anything.
> Student A: But, I get so nervous when there is silence. I guess I do talk a lot—to avoid the quietness. I hate silence, but I guess I'll have to try to cut down on my talking.
> Student B: I can try to help fill in the silent spots so that you don't have to feel that you're the only one responsible for helping our group get something accomplished.

This sharing of information through confrontation allowed both group members to learn something about themselves and to elect to change some of their ways of interacting.

Experiential confrontation: Sharing with another person if there is a discrepancy between the way you see that person and the way she sees herself is known as experiential confrontation. It asks a person to consider another point of view.

—"You say you want to share your load, and yet you don't come prepared for conference."

—"You seem angry with me and you avoid looking at me. Yet, you say you feel fine."

—"You say you want to learn from me, but you don't listen to me. You interrupt me frequently, and you don't look at me when I'm talking."

—"You say you want to develop responsible behavior, and yet you do not come to conference on time either in the morning or in the afternoon."

—"You say that our group is important to your learning, and yet you always address your questions to the teacher."

From these examples, you can see that we are interested in confronting the discrepancies that affect interpersonal style and group participation.

Strength confrontation: This involves pointing out to a person the strengths, abilities or resources that he has but either fails to use or does not use fully.

Student A: You really listen to everyone and make helpful statements afterward. You help to clarify ideas and thoughts, This helps me a lot. I wish, though, that you would do it more often. We really seem to get moving when you help us.

Strength confrontation seems to work effectively. Perhaps this is because it is positive and deals with resources rather than with weaknesses.

Weakness confrontation: This involves pointing out to someone what he or she fails to do or does poorly.

Student B: When you attempt to clarify a point, you tend to go off on a tangent. Often this does not seem at all related to what we are talking about. I get confused and mixed up. Then I want to drop the subject right away because I'm so frustrated. I have to sort it all out later, and it's a lot of extra work.

In this example of weakness confrontation, the speaker described the behavior of the person she was confronting and risked sharing some of her reactions to it. Unfortunately, as often happens with the person being confronted, the student receiving the feedback became defensive. It might have been more helpful if the feedback had been partially a strength confrontation.

Student B: Whenever we get stuck on a point, you work really hard at clarifying it. And you help me to understand the material in more depth. Sometimes, though, you get off on a tangent, and I get confused and mixed up.

If what is being emphasized is almost exclusively a weakness, the odds are that the confrontation will not be effective. The subtle shift in the above example shows how to challenge someone's weakness, but also how to make it at least partially a strength confrontation.

Encouragement to action: This involves identifying the problem and then deciding on a plan of action.

Group of four students:

Student A (to group members): Well, I don't remember any of us doing any gate-keeping (encouraging or supporting each other). That function was certainly lacking in our performance.
Student B: Yes, and a couple of times I really felt it, when I was trying to remember the negative feedback system, and no one tried to help me. I really felt isolated and alone.
Student C: Yes, and I certainly left you hanging out there. I hardly contributed to the discussion at all.
Student D: Well, I talked a lot, but I guess I didn't really listen very much to anyone else. I was busy filling in the answers.
Student A: I was pretty quiet myself. I'll try and talk more.
Student C: Me, too. I'll see if I can help out some the next time.
Student D: I guess we're all going to try harder.

After identifying concrete problems in the interaction of the group members, this group went on to call for action. Some of the action encouraged was more specific than other. "I'll talk more" is more specific than "We're all going to try harder." If the call to action had been generally more specific, however, the group functioning might have improved more rapidly.

While we do not teach confrontation as a skill, we do help students to use it in a healthy manner to resolve conflicts when they arise in a group. The following are helpful hints from Egan[9] for developing a helpful manner in confrontation. We have found these invaluable to use when facing a situation that calls for challenging.

1. First, use the skills of responding with understanding. This helps communication to go more smoothly.
2. Be tentative in order to avoid making confrontation into an accusation.
3. Be clear about why you are confronting someone. This helps to avoid confronting someone from anger and dumping negative emotions on that person.

4. Before confronting someone, earn the right to do so, by being open to receive confrontation yourself. Also try to understand the person you are confronting, and attempt to communicate this understanding to him first.
5. Do not gang up on a person. He may be overwhelmed.
6. Avoid saving up your confrontations to use all at once, or you may end up acting aggresive and hostile.
7. Be specific and concrete. If you are vague, your confrontation is wasted. The person does not really know what you are saying.

These hints provide us with a concrete approach to helping confrontation promote growth rather than be harmful and destructive.

Immediacy. Immediacy "refers to the ability to discuss with another person, directly and mutually, where you stand at the present in your relationship to him or her, and where you see the other person standing in his relationship to you." [9, pp. 235-246].

Student A: I'm really feeling bad. I sense that you and I are not communicating very well and are on edge with each other. I wonder if we can talk about this?

Immediacy is an exercise in mutuality. Self-disclosure in this situation should be related to what is happening between you and the other person, as it is in this example. Immediacy is an invitation to talk about relationship.

An increased familiarity with the communication skills we have just described has enhanced our ability to determine how well students are able to communicate. Not only has our assessment of communication—good or bad—improved, but we can now offer assistance in a concrete manner to those who need it.

Effect of Communication on the Classroom Environment

One of our aims as teachers is to provide an environment that is conducive to fulfilling the individual learning needs of every student. This is a difficult challenge, as each student comes to us with a different background and is at a different stage in both her cognitive and affective development. When we have promoted skillful communication in our conferences, we have succeeded in personalizing the learning environment. The atmosphere is no longer quiet and teacher-centered. It is a constant hum of discussion. Students are exchanging information and experiences that are significant to themselves, helping to clarify issues and sharing feelings. If you listen carefully, you can hear students becoming spontaneously responsible for setting their own goals.

—"I sure need to look that material over again. I thought I knew it."

—"I worked very hard on this section. I feel really good because I had a chance to go over it and explain it here. Now I really understand it. I don't think I'll forget it that easily."

—"I need to be more assertive."

—"I realize I talk too much, and I don't give anyone else a chance. I'm trying very hard now to let everyone else share first, before I do. I'm finding this quite hard. It's easier for me to talk and talk fast."

—"I needed to say something about what was happening. Instead I ran away. Now I'm aggravated at myself. I'm going to talk about it in our group."

—"I have come better prepared."

—"I don't talk enough. I'm not really doing my share. I'm listening and learning. I'm taking but not giving much back."

We are very excited when we listen to students verbalize this kind of awareness of their learning needs and establish their own cognitive and affective goals. Our role then becomes one of acting as resource persons to assist them in fulfilling their goals.

In comparing our previous didactic classroom atmosphere with the present one, we find that there is a great deal more involvement and intimacy among the students. They offer each other understanding, support and caring. In fact, the atmosphere in one particular group offered extensive warmth, support and caring to two students who were having severe academic problems. They were involved in making a decision about whether to withdraw and receive a "W" for the course, or to stay, take the final and receive a probable F or D grade on their transcript. Neither grade is passing. The openness, support and caring of the group members for these students during their difficult time of decision making enabled them to remain as vital parts of the group, through to the end of the semester. During a later discussion of the situation, the failing students each described the support, understanding, and warmth from other group members as having been extremely valuable to them, when at times their academic problems had made them feel depressed and worthless.

Communication skills really make a difference in our reaching. We reach students on a much deeper level of understanding than we have before. They also are able to reach out and touch each other with greater empathy. The whole atmosphere is electric with simultaneous multiple kinds of learning. Where there were once mere classrooms filled with students, there are now productive groups of students self-directing and responsible for their own learning.

GROUP DYNAMICS

Groups are common to all of us, something we all participate in. A group is an association between two or more persons in which there is some sort of interdependent interaction of the members. Interdependence is the core process that renders a group definitive and distinguishes it from a collection or aggregate of independent persons. A group interacts, reacts and modifies. The members affect and are affected by each other.

Interdependence

The basis for interdependence in a group may stem from a common purpose or task (e.g., a nursing staff providing patient care), a shared attribute (e.g., an AA group) or a pattern of interaction that has been established together (e.g., the overprotective mother and the submissive child). As can be seen from the examples, the outcome of group interdependence can be positive or negative. Regardless of outcomes, a collection of people does not constitute a group until they no longer feel the need to act independently when they are together, but feel a desire to share, trust and care about the group as a whole and each of its members as individuals and to accept interdependence as a positive experience. This type of group functioning requires time and direction to establish.

There are many processes that occur along the way toward the development of interdependence. An awareness of these processes affords us an opportunity to observe the dynamics among people as they develop into a group. In Chapter 5, we will discuss the teacher's role in facilitating this development.

Formal and Informal Group Functions

One of the first characteristics of groups that should be considered is that of their function. Groups function on both primary and secondary levels, that is, formally and informally. "A useful way of focusing on this distinction within all groups is to speak about two types of functions that all groups must serve: task-related, or instrumental, functions and member-related, interpersonal functions involving group maintenance"[19, p. 31]. We have found that these two functions must be mutually dependent in order to achieve successful outcomes in post-clinical conferences. The student groups receive a task assignment for the conference. The formal aspect of the function is aimed at carrying out the task and achieving the associated learning objective. The informal aspect involves the way each member relates to the others as persons. Informal functions help maintain group morale, positive feelings among members and a consensus of purpose based on task accomplishment.

Thus there are elements of both the cognitive and the affective in the group learning situation. In order to complete the assigned cognitive task, the feelings of the members must be considered. Discord in informal functions reduces cognitive learning, whereas supportive friendship patterns enhance it[20]. Schmuck found that "student academic performances were conditioned by emotional contents associated with their self-concepts as peers and students, and that these self-concepts were influenced in part by the students' friendship and influence relationships with their classmates" [20, p. 10] . The interpersonal relationships within the group greatly affect the quality and quantity of the cognitive learning that takes place.

Cohesiveness

Another process that occurs in groups is the establishment and maintenance of cohesiveness. This refers to the feelings each of the group members has toward the group as a whole. Cohesiveness embodies a sense of collective and personal belonging. It conveys a sense of security in that each member is important to the whole group, and all members are individually important to each other.

We have seen good development of cohesiveness expressed on self-evaluations of post-clinical conference groups:

—"Our group really worked well together. We all did our part."
—"Sometimes, I didn't understand something, and the group would help me to see it, and they never made me feel put down for not understanding."
—"Everyone shares, no one person carries the load."
—"It's great. When I talk, the group really listens, and then they comment on it or share their experiences or feelings. I really feel good about the group."

Cohesive groups are more goal-directed and productive. The feeling of belonging increases the student's security and satisfaction with herself. The student feels involved with and close to her peers. This kind of positive feeling for self and others frees the student from tension, hostility and self-doubt and allows her to concentrate her energies on the task at hand.

Group Norms

The establishment of group norms is another core process of significance. All groups have group norms. They are the shared expectations or acceptable standards for behavior, attitudes and, perhaps, perceptions of the group members. Norms define what is appropriate and inappropriate behavior for the group members. In this respect, they serve as stabilizers within the group and provide an identifiable limit of behavior for the members to adhere to.

Setting Norms. The success of adherence to group norms appears to rest heavily on two factors. First, groups who are allowed to set their own norms are much more responsive to these norms. While it is important that the teacher lend direction in establishing them, the enforcement of teacher-imposed norms tends to meet with group resistance. Thus the teacher's direction must be subtle and non-threatening. If the teacher wishes to facilitate a standard of democracy, understanding and courtesy, she must demonstrate these behaviors herself.

An example of subtle norm structuring is seen in the attending and responding skills conference referred to earlier in the chapter. The students practice careful listening to what is said, perceiving and discussing the feeling or attitude the speaker conveys. Identifying the content and the feeling facilitates empathic understanding. While the student experiences this as a practice skill early in her group process experience, it serves also as a norm model for her behavior. This norm model may also be applied to patient interaction.

Following the one-to-one attending and responding exercise, the whole student group assembles to discuss their feelings, reactions and difficulties related to the exercise. This type of activity fosters further norm development. The group members can identify what was significant to the listener, what was significant to the speaker. Thus they begin to define what constitutes appropriate behavior, and the norm for verbal interaction begins to emerge. We find a significant modification in attending and responding skills in our post-clinical conferences following practice with this exercise. This behavior also tends to carry over into personal life and to the clinical unit with patient interaction. The students like being carefully attended when they speak, and will respond accordingly when other group members speak. Eventually, member conformity to this type of behavior establishes it as a group norm that is further strengthened by the fact that it is instituted and adopted by the group itself.

Flexibility of Norms. The second factor that affects the successful establishment of group norms is the flexibility of the norms. Narrow limits and rigid norms are frequently broken by group members. Broad norms that allow for individuality, generation of new ideas and modification of group behavior are less threatening and offer a tone of positive encouragement. Narrow limits foster tension among group members. Fear of breaking them with resultant group disapproval or even censorship may escalate anxiety levels to a point where the task-oriented group becomes less productive or nonproductive, and interactive relationships among members begin to deteriorate due to mistrust and fear.

The group's norms must offer enough latitude for its members to feel comfortable and secure within the framework. They must be expansive enough to foster freedom of expression and difference of opinion, but restrictive enough to facilitate task completion and preserve individual rights.

Conformity. Conformity to established norms is controlled by the group. Different groups handle this issue differently. Pressure for adherence to norms may take many forms: Threats, physical restraint or punishment are group pressures more common to family groups, the military and perhaps some classrooms. We have found group pressure to be somewhat more subtle, but usually just as effective.

Most groups reinforce acceptable behavior with praise, verbal agreement and positive nonverbal response: a smile or an assenting nod. The member receiving this type of response feels good. She recognizes that her behavior is acceptable to the group and she gets a feeling of being rewarded for it. Thus she finds that conforming to the group norm is a positive experience for her.

On the other hand, negative group pressure may be brought to bear on the member who does not conform. This may include verbal reproachment, rejection or even ostracism from the group. One of the more common pressures we see is that of exclusion, that is, the group functions around the nonconforming member, relatively oblivious to the member until confrontation or conformity resolves the issue.

An example of this occurred in a group where one member constantly came to pharmacology pre-clinical conference unprepared. She contributed nothing to the group discussion, but took copious notes as the other members shared their information. The group tolerated this behavior for a few weeks, but the mounting tension was visible. Finally, the group began rotating information, so the unprepared member was forced to take a turn and present some information. This heightened her anxiety, a feeling she did not enjoy. On one occasion, she arrived late to conference and found her group engrossed in active discussion with their chairs pulled in a tight, small, closed circle. She got the message: come prepared to share, or don't come into the group.

While this may seem somewhat drastic, it proved to be effective pressure on a group member who was being tacitly resistant to an established group norm by not contributing to group work. The student subsequently began coming prepared and was welcomed again into the group, and her modified behavior was positively reinforced.

Five Aids to Group Process. As stated earlier, norms serve as stabilizers within the group. Through the establishment of norms, the group can institute a pattern of functioning that helps them complete their task. Stanford[22] identifies five areas in which norm establishment is indicated if group process is to develop successfully. They are group responsiblity, responsiveness to others, cooperation, decision making through consensus and confronting problems. There must be identification of and agreement on acceptable individual and group behavior regarding these areas fairly early in the development of group process.

Group Responsibility. One of the first norms the group must develop if it is to be productive is group responsibility. The members must agree to become responsible for their own functioning and to contribute to the group's activities. We have found this often to be a formidable task for our students, who are accustomed to didactic education and formal teacher leadership.

We try to encourage group responsibility early on. Usually during the second or third post-clinical conference of the semester, after initial orientation, we begin to guide the students toward independent functioning in small groups. Typically, following an open discussion with the students regarding the objectives and goals of group process, we will form our student groups. As our clinical faculty/student ratio is one to ten, we usually work with two groups of five students each. The groups are established at random. Usually, we have the students count off by twos—all the ones are in one group, and the twos are in another group. This method is very democratic and facilitates expedient formation of the groups.

The beginning of group responsibility can be facilitated by assigning a simple task that requires a group decision, a decision that formerly was the teacher's prerogative. For example, they are asked to discuss and decide how and when they would like to receive their weekly clinical assignments. Several options are suggested and the groups are informed that they may pursue any original method they feel is workable, but the whole group must agree. Usually, after the task has been explained and questions answered, the groups sit relatively silent, waiting for a teacher's direction. We have found it helpful to leave the room or busy ourselves elsewhere for five or ten minutes to reinforce the understanding that this is a group responsibility, and we are not available for direct supervision or decision making, and to decrease authority-related anxiety. This type of initial approach tends to work well as an introduction to group responsibility.

Responsiveness to others. This second norm relates to the students attending and responding skills. Again, it may be necessary for the teacher to remove herself from the immediate group environment as students may be accustomed to teacher-student discussion rather than student-student discussion. Practice with one-to-one attending and responding, together with group sharing, helps the students develop responsiveness to others.

As the students become more comfortable with group process, they begin to realize that the majority of their learning in the post-clinical conference comes from their peers. While the instructor serves as a reference or resource person, it is the members of the group who actually provide or secure the information necessary for task completion. This realization further reinforces the need for norm development in the areas of responsibility and responsiveness.

Cooperation. This third norm is not always easy to establish, as many students are more familiar with the competitive aspects of the classroom. Cooperation comes from a sense of shared interests, purposes and goals. By comparison, "in a purely cooperative group, any one member's success or failure signifies success or failure for all the others . . .. [I]n a purely competitive group, any one member's success signifies failure (or much reduced success) for the others"[19, p. 27].

There are many obvious benefits derived from group cooperation. Among these are the fostering of attentiveness and greater mutual understanding, and higher quality of work as a result of broader and more varied input. Group cohesiveness, pride in the group, increased self-esteem, plus a general sense of friendliness and well-being are further outcomes of group cooperation.

A simple exercise to foster cooperation involves handing out to each group of five students several (20 to 30) "clues," each on a 3 x 5 card. A clue is a sign, symptom or fact about a patient; some are relevant and some are not. The group members must work with the clues and try to determine the patient's medical diagnosis and nursing needs, and formulate a nursing care plan. As we work with two student groups, we usually give the same clues to each, and compare results between them at the end of the exercise. Competition between groups seems to stimulate greater cooperation within them.

On completion of the exercise, the groups discuss cooperation among them-selves. They try to identify which behaviors were most helpful and which were the least helpful. For instance, one member had suggested the group sit on the floor and spread the clue cards out so that everyone could see them. The rest agreed and found this action helpful. It was interesing to note that within five minutes the other group was also on the floor! Thus cooperation within the group enhances group functioning and productivity. It fosters a greater sense of group identity without which a group cannot function, but merely exists as an aggregate of independent, competitive individuals.

Consensus decision making. Still another group norm is consensus decision making, not to be confused with majority rule. In majority rule, some members (the minority) disagree with the decision but are overruled and must go along with it. Consensus decision making involves consideration of the feelings and needs of each group member.

Consensus, while not always attainable, encourages students to listen carefully and understand the meaning of communication. All thoughts and opinions of-fered must be considered. The individual group members may have to reconsider their opinions, perhaps alter them or compromise. Consensus decision making requires an open mind; mistrust, competition and insecurity all serve to hinder the process. It allows for ventilation of all ideas and feelings regarding the task at hand. The input of all the group members affords each individual the opportunity to broaden her perceptions and expand her knowledge, thereby providing more information with which to make a more thoughtful decision.

We have found that groups that have continual difficulties with consensus decision making have also demonstrated problems with cooperation, a low level of cohesiveness and narrow rigid norms that do not allow for openness and ex-pression of divergent opinions. A decision from consensus is one that all members can support and feel comfortable with. This type of decision making requires well-developed listening skills and an empathic, mature attitude on the part of each group member.

Confronting problems. A major stumbling block to consensus decision making is frequently a group's inability to confront problems within the group. Confrontation in a group usually requires that the members stop all activity regarding the current task and take a long look at where each member stands and why. It is important for each to try to verbalize the problem as she sees it and explain exactly what type of behavior she sees going on within the group. If the members are able to describe existing behaviors that are detrimental to the group's productivity, they can pursue the reasons or motivations behind the behaviors. It is necessary to analyze and define what is happening that is causing conflict before the group can attempt conflict resolution.

Avoidance of confrontation is detrimental to group process. The tendency to skirt the problem issue or to tolerate it often leads to anxiety, suppressed anger and perhaps some form of openly expressed hostility. Some members may withdraw verbally from the group, others may become angry and overbearing. Group productivity slows down or ceases entirely until conflict is resolved through confrontation.

Since our groups are basically task-oriented, the problem-solving approach to conflict seems to be the best means for confronting it, and one that is familiar to nursing students. The first action on the group's part is to acknowledge the existence of a problem. Then data collection and assessment may take place. Each member is allowed to express her feelings openly and to define what she thinks the problem is. The use of feedback and feeling identification is often helpful to clarify each member's feelings and to enhance understanding. Open lines of communication, honesty, empathy and respect are the basic tools for conflict resolution.

An example of active group confrontation occurred when one of our post-clinical conference groups, consisting of five student nurses, began to deteriorate. Student A was a rather outspoken, dominating person. As the self-appointed group leader, she initiated and controlled all discussion. She was usually well prepared and often corrected or criticized other group members during discussion. She felt her behavior was assertive; the group viewed it as aggressive and responded accordingly. Student B, an academically weak student, withdrew out of intimidation. Student C tried hard to keep up with Student A, but often found herself involved in a game of one-upmanship. Student D fought openly with Student A. Student E, an older student, assumed the role of peacemaker and attempted to maintain the group.

At midsemester, each group member was asked to fill out an evaluation form on the progress of their group including strengths, weaknesses, and areas for improvement. They were then asked to share their feelings with the other members.

Student A: Well, I really love group process. I get to speak out and help others in the group.
Student E: Yes, I like it too, but I think maybe everyone doesn't have as much opportunity to participate as they might.
Student A: Well, no one's stopping them!

Student C: Sometimes when I'm trying to say something, I am interrupted and then I lose my train of thought.

Student B: Yes, that's annoying. It makes you feel like what you're saying isn't important.

Student D: Right! And the point of group process is supposed to be to allow everyone input. [To Student A] : Every one of us wants to speak out and be listened to. We should all be able to share our ideas.

Student E: Then perhaps under improvement, we should try to be more democratic.

Student B: And more courteous.

Student A: Well, I know sometimes I'm a little pushy, but sometimes I feel like everyone isn't prepared, and I have to carry the group. [Looks toward Student B.]

Student E: Well, we can all work on being better prepared for conferences so that we all have something significant to contribute.

Student C: Okay, that's good. I really like to hear what other people think; it helps me to understand better.

Student A: It's okay with me, too.

The group members were able to express their feelings regarding a problem the group had encountered in a nonaggressive, positive way through the use of a simple evaluation tool and the problem-solving approach. Two suggestions emerged: one, that democracy and courtesy be extended to all members at all times; and two, that all members assume the responsibility of coming well prepared to clinical conference. Following this confrontation, the group functioned more productively, although a bit tentatively for the next few sessions. Through confrontation, new and more acceptable behavioral norms were established; these served better to meet the members' needs.

Conflict and conflict resolution are often strengthening processes. Cooperation and a responsibility for the well-being of the group are factors that motivate a group toward conflict resolution. Confrontation of problems is a healthy sign in group development, even though the process usually evolves as a result of destructive conflict. Once a problem has been confronted and resolved, a norm for dealing with group problems has been established. The members then know how better to handle future problems and have a behavioral guideline.

STAGES IN GROUP DEVELOPMENT

It is naive to believe that one can bring together a collection of people and expect that by calling them a group, they will in fact behave like one and function with the required skills. A group is like an individual, it must move through developmental stages to become a productive working unit. The group must deal with the problems or tasks that occur in each stage before progressing on to the next. Schmuck[20] states that the stages in group development are sequential and successive, and that problems occurring in one will be handled in a manner established in a prior stage. These stages provide growth guidelines, through which the group passes as it develops its formal and informal relationships.

As in human development, the group may find itself arrested at one stage and unable to progress to the next. For instance, if the group has not established a working norm for cooperation, it will not be able effectively to carry out any assigned activity that required cooperative effort. Some groups never develop openness and trust, and therefore remain arrested in an early stage of group development. Helping the group identify its stage of development and what type of behavior is occurring to cause its lack of progress may assist in bringing about the necessary confrontation and resolution. Trial and error, evaluation and adaptation are frequently the methods used to accomplish each developmental stage.

The stages in group development are not absolute, that is, characteristics of each stage can be found in successive ones. While an early stage may concern itself almost wholly with orientation of group members to each other, this process continues throughout the entire life of the group.

Each group must be allowed to progress at its own rate and in its own pattern. We often find that although we work with two clinical conference groups that have been exposed to similar theoretical and clinical experiences and are assigned the same group activity, they seldom are at the same developmental stage at any point in time. In fact, each one usually handles the assignment differently, according to their level of developmental growth and group maturity.

Before discussing the actual stages of group development, it is important to comment on the teacher's role. The teacher facilitates the progression of the group through each developmental stage. As group process depends greatly on learned behavior and acquisition of communication skills, some knowledgeable guidance and direction are necessary. The teacher's influence is often vital to group productivity, but the method of influence is one of facilitation of events and outcomes rather than direct didactic intervention. In Chapter 5, we will discuss the teacher's role in detail, presenting examples of facilitative techniques.

Stanford[21, p. 27] describes "five stages through which a group would ideally move when the teacher intervenes to maximize their group development." The five stages are: orientation, establishing norms, coping with conflict, productivity and termination.

Orientation

The orientation stage is the early period of group formation during which the student attempts to define her position and role with regard to setting and circumstance. Questions that must be answered in this stage are: What is going to happen here? Who are these other people and what is my relationship to them? What is expected of me?

Initially the student is anxious about presenting a poor image. She desires a secure place in the peer group. There is often a great deal of stress, with fear of rejection or ridicule. The student acquires information regarding teacher and peer expectations and course requirements during the orientation stage.

Schmuck[20] cites the establishment of acceptance, inclusion, membership and trust as the developmental tasks of the first stage in group development. The main theme involves testing the reactions of others. The student learns in this stage to deal with lack of familiarity and situational anxiety. Desired outcomes of the orientation stage include: acquaintance with group members, understanding the function of group process and a beginning involvement and identification that will foster a feeling of security.

This is the time of initial opening of the channels of communication. While the student is usually rather tentative in early communication, she finds that she is put more at ease as she gathers more information and this, in turn, encourages further communication. It is vitally important for the teacher to provide the means for the student to receive all the necessary information she requires to allow her enough security to begin to function within the group. The orientation stage is a time for exploring, questioning, defining, learning and evaluating the new educational situation.

Establishing Norms

If the group has passed successfully through the orientation stage, the members are usually more relaxed and open, and a sense of trust and cohesiveness has developed. Stage 2 usually centers on organizing the group into a productive functioning unit. There is sometimes a power struggle of sorts regarding group leadership. Decisions on organization, definition of roles, values and common communication are made during this stage.

The group sets behavior standards for itself and determines how it might best accomplish its formal and informal functions. The goal of Stage 2 is for the group to become self-directing, to establish responsibility for itself as a functioning unit and for its own learning. This goal must be accomplished without stifling the independence or individuality of any of the members. Thus accommodation and adaptation become characteristics of Stage 2.

The establishment of norms is often an extremely difficult stage. Success seems dependent on the level of communication that has been reached. Shared expectations and feelings, mutual trust and respect foster the decision-making process regarding acceptable group norms. We start to see improvement of communication skills during this stage, as the students attempt to establish a valuable, workable group protocol. If communication fails, the group will fragment into cliques whose members share common interests and values. Group productivity is greatly diminished in this instance, and the mastery of Stage 2 developmental level is arrested.

The teacher's role in Stage 2 is to facilitate student participation and communication. Active communication will usually foster the development of high group involvement and interest. When members care about the group, the establishment and maintenance of norms becomes desirable to them.

Coping with Conflict

The conflict stage is generally considered an inevitability by experts in group dynamics. It occurs when a group that has been productive and cohesive starts to show signs of increasing bickering, arguing or outright hostility. This behavior may be directed at other group members or at the teacher.

If the students have successfully completed Stage 2 (norm development), they have defined an acceptable way to deal with confrontation, and the fear of confrontation should be minimized. Conflicts that may have been suppressed are now permitted to emerge. The conflict is probably not new at all, but was previously controlled or ignored because of earlier inability to deal with confrontation.

As communication skills progress, there is more widespread involvement of group members bringing a greater diversity of opinions into the discussion, and their differences in goals, values and personal feelings surface. The group intimacy and cohesiveness that have developed afford the group members the courage to speak out their convictions. This may result in conflict.

Sometimes the conflict is directed toward the teacher. This is often expressed as a challenge for more independence or a rebellion against teacher leadership. We have frequently had a group tell us, "We know you assigned the task this way, but we all decided we prefer to do it another way." This is the true test of the teacher! While we have been encouraging sharing of feelings and opinions, it is somewhat of a jolt when our well thought-out assignments are challenged, altered or voted down. When this occurs, it is the teacher who must serve as a role model demonstrating proper handling of conflict with an objective, accepting approach, allowing free expression of opinion regarding the problem.

Many experts believe that without conflict there is no personal growth. When everyone in the group is in agreement, there is no need to examine one's own behavior. Conflict can be positive in that it exposes differing feelings. It enhances understanding by allowing the group members a closer look at each other and at themselves.

Guidance in the proper handling of conflict may be necessary, or the classroom could become a virtual battlefield. Reinforcement of previously learned communication skills—active listening, empathic understanding and regard for established norms—all aid in guiding a group in conflict through open, problem-solving confrontation. It is best for the teacher to accept and anticipate conflict as an inevitable stage as the group moves toward independent functioning and maturity. With acknowledgment and acceptance of this, the teacher can concentrate on helping the students learn constructive ways to deal with conflict.

Productivity

The productivity stage is the ultimate goal of group development. In this stage, the group functions as a productive unit in both formal and informal activities. Task accomplishment is high and interpersonal relationships are strong. Although problems still arise, the group knows how to deal with conflict constructively.

It is important during this stage that a balance be maintained between the group's attention to cognitive tasks and to interpersonal relationships. If too much emphasis is placed on one, the other usually suffers. A comment we have had on student evaluations has verified this point:

—Our group worked great. We all got along very well and really cared about each other, but sometimes we'd go off on a personal tangent, and we would not finish our assignment."

Concentration on one area more than the other is expected and acceptable, and should only be a concern if the group becomes involved in one area to the total exclusion of the other. Usually, if imbalance occurs in our groups, it is in the direction of interpersonal relationships, and task productivity starts to slide. At this point, teacher intervention is necessary to bring the problem to light and help the group determine how it might again achieve balance between its formal and informal functions.

Termination

The fifth and final stage of group development is termination. The students have always known their group would eventually terminate, but there are various activities that can make the ending valuable.

Group members should have an opportunity to share their feelings about the dissolution of the group, how being a part of a group has affected them personally, their growth and their communication skills. In the termination stage, the members have an opportunity to tell each other what they learned from each other. We usually ask them to evaluate the effects of group process skills on their interactions with patients and their acquisition of cognitive knowledge. The group usually evaluates how they functioned as a group throughout the semester, pointing out strengths and weaknesses.

In all, this stage offers an opportunity to evaluate their achievement in relation to purpose and goals, and a chance to say goodbye to a group caring and sharing peers, helpers, teachers, learners and friends.

ACTIVITY PHASES OF A GROUP SESSION

All individual group sessions are composed of various activity phases, during which specific tasks must be accomplished. Stanford[21] discusses three distinct phases: warm-up, the activity phase, and the integration phase. We have found that recognition and acceptance of these three phases has helped us guide our students to more productive work. The first and third are of critical importance, as the warm-up phase allows the students opportunity to get in the mood for the group task, and the integration phase allows them time to put it all together and evaluate outcomes.

Warm-up Phase

The warm-up phase occurs during the first several minutes of our post-clinical conference group sessions. Its purpose is to allow the students time to separate themselves from previous activity, clear their minds of immediate past experience, receive directions regarding their task assignment for the session and tune in to the present situation.

We usually allow five to fifteen minutes of our post-clinical conference hour for warm-up, although this varies according to the circumstances. Our students come to post-clinical conference directly from the clinical unit and usually need an opportunity to ventilate about their clinical expereince. Invariably, someone will have been involved with a new procedure, cared for a special patient or perhaps had a bad day and will want to discuss it with the group. Occasionally, a clinical situation discussed in the warm-up phase will be extremely pertinent, or of such interest to the group that discussion of the situation with all its ramifications and nursing indications becomes the focus of the session. That tends to be the exception rather than the rule; however, students do need to talk about their clinical experiences before they can put them aside and concentrate on the task for the session.

The second part of the warm-up phase involves giving the students their group task assignment. Specific objectives and directives are given and any questions regarding the assignment are answered. The students then gather any materials or notes they might need and settle down to their group activity.

Activity Phase

The activity phase usually involves two stages: "getting ready" and "getting it together." The students seem to require a "getting ready" stage in which they can present their feelings and ideas regarding the assignment and its relevance to them. This type of activity helps personalize the task and the outcome. During this stage, the students usually review the task and decide how they want to go about accomplishing it. Once the format for task completion has been established, the group commences the actual work.

It is important to recognize that the students will not begin productive activity until they have passed through the warm-up phase and "getting ready" stage. Disruption, inappropriate talking or excessive physical activity that prolong the time it takes to get to work usually indicate that the students have had an inadequate warm-up phase and have not passed successfully out of it yet. The time it takes a group to accomplish this varies considerably. Typically we find with our two groups that one seems to be able to get into the assignment fairly readily, while the other needs more time to discuss the assignment and "psych" themselves into a productive frame of mind. One of the most positive aspects of group process is the flexibility it affords students to progress at their own pace and in their own way.

The last stage of the activity phase involves putting all the information together to come out with a consolidated whole. Conclusions are drawn and pertinent points further clarified. The group then has a final product as the result of its endeavors.

Integration Phase

Integration is the final phase, wherein information is shared and evaluated. This phase also involves discussing the individual and professional significance of the assignment.

We usually allow both groups to come together into one large group for the last five to ten minutes of the conference hour. We review the objectives of the assignment and ask the students to share their information and outcomes. Sharing information contributes to the students' knowledge pool and often clarifies many points that may not have been resolved satisfactorily.

We then ask the individual members to share their thoughts and feelings regarding the significance of the assignment to them personally. Comments range from, "I learned a lot; this will really help me with my patient care," to "I don't think I got much out of this conference." We thankfully have received less of the latter type of comment since we started using group process.

The integration phase is vital to the students in that they can see their accomplishment and its relevance to themselves. It also affords the teacher the opportunity to receive information regarding the educational value of the assignment from the student's point of view.

These activity phases also are adaptable, on a larger scale, to a typical clinical day. We can consider the pre-clinical conference as the warm-up phase. From this perspective, the half-hour pre-clinical conference allows the students an opportunity to review their patient assignments for the day. This allows for input from group members regarding the care plan and how it might be optimally effective.

The clinical focus for the day is presented by the instructor and discussed with the students. The clinical focus correlates with the classroom content presented that week as do the clinical patient assignments. Thus, during the clinical day warm-up phase, the students prepare themselves mentally and emotionally for their clinical experience. They are familiarized with the learning objective for the day and have had an opportunity to correlate verbally the objective with the clinical assignment; this lends direction to their learning expereince.

The activity phase of the clinical day consists of actual patient care. The first stage—"getting ready"—includes receiving report from a staff nurse, reviewing the patient's chart and care plan, and the initial introductory patient encounter. The second stage—"getting it together"—encompasses all the subsequent patient care or patient-related activities in which the student participates for the remainder of the assigned clinical time period.

The integration phase consists of post-clinical conference wherein the day's activities are shared and evaluated. This activity correlated directly with the focus for the day, which was presented in the pre-clinical conference.

In this chapter, we have presented the basics of group process as we practice it. We feel the process itself is an effective, confluent and dynamic teaching method and fosters positive teacher-student communication, allowing for intellectual and personal growth on the parts of both. In Chapter 5, we will pursue the role of the teacher as a facilitator of group process.

REFERENCES

1. Anthony, W., and Carkhuff, R. *The Art of Health Care: A Handbook of Psychological First Aid Skills.* Amherst, Mass.: Human Resource Development, 1976.
2. Bates, M., and Johnson, C. *Group Leadership.* Denver, Colo.: Love, 1972.
3. Benjamin, A. *The Helping Interview.* Boston: Houghton Mifflin, 1969.
4. Brill, N. *Teamwork.* Philadelphia: Lippincott, 1976.
5. Brill, N. *Working with People: The Helping Process.* Philadelphia: Lippincott, 1978.
6. Carkhuff, R., and Pierce, R. *The Art of Helping III: Trainer's Guide.* Amherst, Mass.: Human Resource Development, 1977.
7. Clark, C. *The Nurse as Group Leader.* New York: Springer, 1977.
8. Egan, G. *The Skilled Helper.* Monterey, Calif.: Brooks/Cole, 1975.
9. Egan, G. *You and Me: The Skills of Communicating and Relating to Others.* Monterey, Calif.: Brooks/Cole, 1977.
10. Gazda, G.; Asbury, F.; Balzer, F.; Childers, W.; and Walters, R. *Human Relations Development: A Manual for Educators.* Boston: Allyn and Bacon, 1977.
11. Gazda, G.; Walters, R.; and Childers, W. *Human Relations Development: A Manual for Health Sciences.* Boston: Allyn and Bacon, 1975.
12. Glasser, W. *Reality Therapy.* New York: Harper and Row, 1965.
13. Lifton, W. *Groups: Facilitating Individual Growth and Societal Change.* New York: Wiley, 1972.
14. Marram, G. *The Group Approach in Nursing Practice.* St. Louis: Mosby, 1973.
15. Miller, J. *Humanizing the Classroom: Models of Teaching Affective Education.* New York: Praeger, 1976.
16. McLuhan, M., and Fiore, Q. *The Medium Is the Massage.* New York: Random House, 1967.
17. Patterson, C. *Humanistic Education.* Englewood Cliffs, N.J.: Prentice-Hall, 1973.
18. Rogers, C. *Freedom to Learn.* Columbus, Ohio: Charles E. Merrill, 1969.
19. Sampson, E., and Marthas, M. *Group Process for the Health Professions.* New York: Wiley, 1977.
20. Schmuck, R., and Schmuck, P. *Group Process in the Classroom.* Dubuque, Iowa: Wm. C. Brown, 1971.
21. Stanford, G. *Developing Effective Classroom Groups.* New York: Hart, 1977.
22. Stanford, G., and Roark, A. *Human Interaction in Education.* Boston: Allyn and Bacon, 1974.

CHAPTER 5

The Role of the Teacher

The role of the teacher is an extremely influential one. The teacher has an effect, either positive or negative, on a student's affective and cognitive growth. If she is able to develop a good relationship with a student, the effect she has will probably be positive. Unfortunately, if her relationship with a student is poor, her effect may well be negative. The kind of relationship a teacher establishes with students is stressed as being important because it sets the tone for all other interactions that occur in the classroom. Stanford and Roark[27, p. viii] maintain that "the chief functions of teachers are to engage in interpersonal relationships which are healthy and growth-producing and to provide environments which favor this type of interaction for students."

Carkhuff[7] supports the concept that the teacher-student relationship is crucial to learning. He sees it as being analagous to a counselor-counselee relationship, as both are helping situations. The factors that were identified as being essential in helping relationships are the same as those that were first cited by Rogers[13] : empathy (understanding), congruence (genuineness) and nonjudgmental, warm personal regard (respect).

Carkhuff and Berenson[8] review and cite research that provides strong indications that the quality of relationships determines whether or not they will be helpful or harmful. If the level of empathy, respect and genuineness is too low in a helping relationship such as teaching, the person being helped (taught) will begin to function at a lower level, both cognitively and affectively. Thus the student can actually be harmed rather than helped. The concept of causing harm to students is relatively new to us. We find it to apply just as strongly in nursing as in any other area of education.

This concept has even greater ramifications when applied to student-student relationships. To us, this means that we as teachers have a definite responsibility for fostering a good relationship between ourselves and students and also among the students, in order to create an environment in which healthy, positive and productive cognitive and affective growth can occur.

This chapter considers factors that will assist a teacher in fulfilling these responsibilities.

STYLES OF LEADERSHIP

There are essentially three categories of leadership styles, separate and distinct in their qualities and in their effects on cognitive and affective learning. Probably no teacher can easily be placed in any one category, but a discussion of each style and its differing effects on classroom learning is pertinent. The three styles to consider are democratic, autocratic and laissez-faire [24, pp. 26-43].

Analysis of the basis of interpersonal influence is helpful to understanding the differences between the styles. Another term for interpersonal influence is power. Schmuck and Schmuck[24, p. 28] review a useful set of categories concerning power or influence:

1. Expert power: how much expert knowledge a person is credited with having
2. Referent power: the degree of closeness others feel toward a person, how much they identify with that person
3. Reward power: the degree to which others view an individual as having the ability to give rewards
4. Coercive power: the degree to which someone is viewed as being able to punish others
5. Legitimate power: the feeling of others that a person has a right to be influential

The appearance of these five bases of influence vary with a teacher's style of leadership. The least effective categories are legitimate, reward and coercive, as they do not contribute to the development of helpful relationships. These are usually given to a teacher by the profession so that control may be maintained in the classroom. Successfully influential or powerful teachers, however, are able to develop additional bases of power, such as referent or expert, with their students. These aid in fostering positive relationships.

DEMOCRATIC LEADERSHIP

The democratic leader bases her power on the students' identifying with her and, to some extent, on having expertise. She does not keep this power for herself, however, but distributes it throughout the group so that increasingly more of the groups' functions are performed by members, rather than by herself. Thus power and responsibility are shared. This kind of leadership creates a climate in which "members can openly express themselves, share their diversity without fear of rejection or excessive conflict, explore their different skills and talents, build upon these in accomplishing their mutual tasks"[23].

The democratic style facilitates active participation of group members in decision making, creating and evaluating policies, looking at alternatives and taking action. The leader's efforts are directed toward manipulating the process. This includes defining the task, suggesting materials to use and serving as a resource person. She also encourages the use of consensus in decision making, helping the group to evaluate its functioning by supporting spontaneous shifts in direction and methods that emerge from within the group that all members agree are in line with established norms. In no way does this type of leader manipulate the individual. "Control of others, no matter how well-intentioned, reduces human beings to the status of things"[28]. Instead, a deomocratic style fosters actualizing of individual student interests and potential; often this is accomplished spontaneously through a group process approach.

The results of this style of leadership as they apply to nursing education are as follows:

1. Students display a high degree of enthusiasm, considerable involvement in and commitment to their work and their group. Motivation is not a problem.

2. Members usually experience satisfaction at having participated in producing a product of high quality (such as getting all the answers correct on a group pharmacology quiz).

3. Cohesiveness, a sense of comradeship and good morale develop.

4. Members become personally responsible and take initiative. They work effectively even when the leader is late or absent. When the instructor arrives, post-clinical conference groups are usually already at work sharing their experience or working on a previously assigned task.

5. Group members learn leadership skills and behavior. Leadership becomes diffused throughout the group, shared at one time or another by all.

This style of leadership is important to cultivate if a teacher is to develop a humanistic approach in the classroom.

Autocratic Leadership

The autocratic style of leadership is leader-centered rather than member-centered. The leader's power is based mostly on legitimacy and coercion and to some extent, on her use of rewarding the students[24, p. 29]. This type of leader makes virtually all of the group's decisions, and gives specific directions as to what the work will be and how it will be accomplished. An autocratic leader feels that she knows best; that her main task is to convince others of the correctness of her own views. Frequently, she will stifle disagreement within the group unless it helps her to achieve her own goals. She tends to be secretive in her dealings with members, believing that members should be prevented from knowing too much. "Keeping members in the dark about what the goals are and what the relation is between present activities and these goals is a typical picture of autocratic leaders. Such people are proficient at covering over issues that might thwart achievement of their own ends for the group. The group for them is not a locus of human resources that need to be tapped, but a means of accomplishing personal goals"[23, p. 195].

As the focus of the group, the autocratic leader tends to foster excessive dependency. No action can be performed or decision made without her. Although she may be a warm and friendly person, she sends out a basic message that says "my way is best." This person will have difficulty using confluent techniques such as group process that facilitate self-actualizing growth in students, because this is opposite to her interest in convincing people her way is the right way.

The results of this style of leadership are as follows:

1. The class members do not grow into a cohesive group. Morale is low.

2. Few new ideas or innovations develop, as members fail to function independently.

3. There may be much resentment and bitterness over having to submit to the rule of the leader. Members may revolt and overthrow the leader. Much energy can be expended in this manner rather than in more productive learning.

4. Feelings of irritability, anger and apathy may predominate. Resistance to the work may develop.

5. The individual members do not take on responsibility for the work. Productivity may be high, but the leader's constant surveillance and supervision are required to keep it that way.

This style of leadership is not the kind that is needed in nursing education, where the development of responsibility, accountability, independence, initiative and cooperation in students are valued.

Laissez-Faire Leadership

The laissez-faire leader abdicates power and performs no legitimate leadership behavior. This leadership style is neither member-centered nor leader-centered. It is rather a non-centered style [24, p. 29].

The laissez-faire leader simply lets things alone to develop as they will. She remains apart from any active involvement in the group. She does not attempt to engage members in discussions or to facilitate member involvement and participation; she does not even take total responsibility in a didactic manner. Instead she tends to let things drift. As a result, clear goals for the group are not established, decisions are not made and ongoing evaluation of group process is missing [23, p. 196]. According to Sampson and Marthas [23], people adopting this style of leadership seem to be distrustful of authority. Unfortunately, the results of such a style tend to be nonproductive. There is confusion and nonfunctioning among the students. Energy is spent on frustration and unrest, or the students may turn to an autocratic member of the group for directive leadership. The group will probably not become a cohesive unit.

The results of this style of leadership are as follows:

1. Members are frustrated and look for someone or something to blame for their frustrations. Scapegoating is a frequent occurrence.

2. There is apathy, low morale and minimal interest in the task or in the group.

3. Productivity is low. The work itself tends to be inefficient and sloppy.

4. Members lack a feeling of group cohesiveness and personal concern for each other.

5. Members are not trained in communication or leadership skills, and there is minimal involvement of students with each other. Each student is more involved with her own activities.

This style of leadership does not offer to students an approach that stimulates learning, either cognitive or affective. It certainly does not provide the kind of confluent stimulus that enhances growth toward self-actualization. It turns its back to task functions as well as to interpersonal functions.

In looking at the styles of leadership, it seems clear that using the democratic style in teaching is more conducive to fostering confluent education. Although there may be circumstances in which a clearly defined line of authority is necessary, for the most part a democratic approach seems better suited for nursing education. Certainly, the democratic teacher will need to be flexible in her management of the learning process, to enable selection of the approach that will best fit the circumstances.

According to Sampson and Marthas[23] the skills that are required for democratic leadership are more demanding and complex than those required for the other styles. No particular skills are required for the uninvolvement of laissez-faire leadership, while only a good sense of the leader's own position and ability to persuade others are necessary for autocratic leadership. More skills are essential for democratic leadership, however. A person must: (1) basically work with group process, (2) adopt a problem-solving approach and facilitate student involvement in it and (3) be willing to treat members as responsible participants and resource people for group action. A democratic teacher must be willing to change her ideas so that she is no longer concerned with personally winning or not losing a point. She must involve group members in discussion and decision making and help them explore, examine and evaluate their own ideas and suggestions.

THE TEACHER AS A FACILITATOR

Competence in a variety of roles enhances the teacher's ability to manage group process to facilitate both cognitive and affective growth of nursing students. These roles include serving as a role model, observer, group participant and resource person.

Teacher As Model

Appropriate modeling by a teacher can be helpful in assisting students to learn desired affective behavior to use when dealing with herself, or when interacting with other students. Patterson[21] states that although modeling may not be the only way, it is probably the most effective way of teaching, especially if combined with some explanation. He goes on to say[21, p. 165] that, "If a teacher is not the kind of person he is trying to teach the students to be, no matter what he does, he cannot teach this. But he will teach whatever he is, whether he is aware of it or intends to or not."

Modeling is currently claimed as a behaviorist method of teaching, although it has been in existence as a way of teaching from the time of primitive societies. In fact, most of us are familiar with the obvious examples of modeling that occur when adult behavior is imitated by young children.

Behaviorists explain that imitation of a model as a form of learning works because it is reinforcing[19]. The reinforcement may come from as many as three different sources. The first one involves direct reinforcement from the model or teacher. The second stems from the consequences of the imitated behavior; this is true especially if the behavior is socially acceptable and leads to the attainment of a goal, both of which bring positive rewards. The third source of reinforcement is a vicarious one, by which the student derives second-hand satisfaction from imitating the model. The imitator assumes that the model does something because she receives some reward or pleasure from what she is doing; thus by carrying out the same behavior, the imitator will also receive the reward that the model receives.

Lefrancois[19, p. 301] indicates that "the greatest advantage that learning by imitation has over other forms of learning is that it provides a complete behavioral sequence for the learner." The need for trial and error learning or for successive approximations is lessened or eliminated. The learner has a model whose behavior she can first observe and then imitate, ultimately experiencing reward for her behavior.

Modeling allows for the learning of complex patterns of behavior as wholes. This can be especially helpful in regard to social behaviors; particularly for learning the complex aspects represented by empathy, respect and genuineness [21, p. 165]. It is difficult if not impossible to teach these through an entirely didactic approach. Although experiential learning through the use of diad and triad role playing is valuable, the most effective way in which a teacher can teach understanding, respect, warmth and genuineness is to demonstrate these qualities herself. The student then not only has a model of appropriate affective behavior to imitate, as a recipient of that behavior she knows firsthand how it feels to experience that kind of behavior. She then is able to imitate the model she had perceived in diad and triad role-playing situations, in her interactions with other members of her group and ultimately with her patients.

Teacher as Observer

The teacher in group process needs to be an informed observer to gather information about the functioning of the group. Ultimately, this role makes possible appropriate intervention to facilitate group development and productivity and to help students evaluate their present situations and future possibilities.

To be an observer, a teacher must be able to view herself and the group with objectivity. She has to develop perspective from a distance. If she remains a full participant, it becomes difficult for her to see just what is going on. She must maintain a delicate balance of being inside the group in order fully to understand and appreciate what is being said and experienced by group members, yet also be outside looking in, to view the interactions objectively.

Earlier we discussed in detail group process dynamics and communication, which are necessary if the teacher is to be an informed observer. We need also to concentrate on what knowledge she needs in order to evaluate the growth and development of individual members within the group and their interrelationships and the effects of her own interactions on the group.

Observations of Group Members.   An informed teacher/observer bases her observations of the individual on a Gestalt holistic conceptual frame-work. She avoids concentrating her observations on the cognitive contributions of the group members. She works at viewing the feelings and values being expressed by each member. To accomplish this, she will need to sharpen her listening skills so that she can pick up not only surface content, but also meanings and implications of what is being said.

To add yet another dimension, she needs to observe students' perceptions of themselves and their environment. Behavior is said to be a function of life space. In other words, we behave in terms of the world as we perceive and experience it, rather than in terms of its more objective features[23]. This means the teacher must understand each member's awareness of her own situation and how she is perceiving the group experience. The teacher must make a concerted effort to hear from the individual's point of view and to see the situation in that person's terms, and avoid hearing and seeing from her own frame of reference. Observations that are tempered with understanding of the students' perspective make a firm basis for valuable personalized intervention.

Another area for concentration of teacher observations is the relationships among group members. Again, the foundation for the teacher's observations is basically the Gestalt concept of holism. It is also helpful, however, to add to that basic foundation some understanding of systems theory. They are compatible with each other, and together provide the teacher with a slightly broader conceptual framework for understanding her observations of both the interdependence of the individuals and the dynamics of group process itself.

Very simply, Gestalt theory offers us a holistic understanding of humans as being one with the environment, each influencing the other. In other words, to understand the behavior of an individual within a group, a teacher must have an awareness of what is happening in the whole group. A knowledge of systems theory provides this. Systems theory offers an explanation and a guide for observing what is happening within the whole group, which ultimately influences the behavior of each individual member.

A group is like a system[23], comprised of elements or parts, which are the individual members. The elements of any system are joined together by a relationship of interdependence, as are the members of a group. Whatever happens to one element in a system has consequences for others. Because of their interdependence, the behavior of one group member is linked intimately with the behavior of all other members.

The meaning of this interdependence is clearer when coupled with the concept that a system or group is always striving for dynamic equilibrium or balance. When something happens to change the behavior of one member, the dynamic equilibrium of the group may be upset. This change can threaten the stability of the group and may be resisted by it. If it occurs despite the resistance, it means that a corresponding change in the behavior of other group members must occur to compensate for the initial change in behavior of the one member. This compensation is essential to retain or reestablish dynamic equilibrium. The teacher who manages group process will find it helpful to be able to identify these compensating changes. This information combined with her observations of members' perceptions and feelings will greatly enhance her holistic understanding of the members, thereby personalizing and increasing the depth of her interventions.

Effects of Teacher Interaction. In addition to her observations, a teacher must also be attentive to current group process and to the fact she is a part of it. The focus of the group's interaction needs to be on the present, and not on past or forthcoming events, with emphasis on options, choices and reactions that the teacher and group members are currently experiencing. The teacher keeps her comments relative to the present, thus setting the tone for the rest of the group. As she observes, experiences and thinks in terms of the here and now, she needs to be in touch with her own feelings, conscious of what in the present experience has precipitated them, and ready to express them if this would be appropriate and helpful.

The teacher must continually work at observing the effects of her interaction with the group. Were her comments really appropriate to the situation, helping to facilitate the discussion or decision making? Or did interaction decrease and the process flounder? If she gave feedback to the group, was the response resistance and defensive anger, or willingness to accept and use? If it was the former, was the feedback really accurate, or could there have been a problem with her observations, or perhaps with the way in which the feedback was offered? If the group accepted the intervention and went on, chances are that the teacher's observations were accurate, her assessments correct and her methods of intervention based on them were helpful.

To summarize, the teacher as observer gathers information, sorts and discriminates it, assesses the group situation and intervenes appropriately as a participant. She next observes the effects of her intervention and evaluates it accordingly.

Teacher as Participant.

The teacher's ability to be an effective participant in the group is based on her functions as an accurate observer. She must offer concrete, behavioral feedback to members individually, or to the group as a whole. Sometimes the teacher may also participate by sharing her own ideas on and reactions to what she is currently experiencing. This must be done sparingly, however, to avoid assuming the role of didactic teacher and taking control of the group.

The feedback that the teacher offers provides the individual with information about her behavior as it is perceived by another person and the group with information about its ongoing deliberations and interactions. It makes students conscious of those behaviors that open communication and points out those that oppose it. It helps members to process their feelings and reactions to the group, thereby facilitating the growth and development of the members as individuals and the group as a unit.

Feedback for Patterns of Behavior that Help or Hinder Communication.

Questions. Questions inhibit communication. Despite this, asking questions is a generally accepted way of trying to communicate. The majority of group members usually depend heavily on them. Awareness that questions control the responder in a subtle way is only dimly perceived by most people. The teacher may often meet with resistance and impatience when she asks a member to abandon her traditional way of controlling others by asking questions and to substitute in its place a clear "I" statement telling what she feels or thinks, i.e., "I feel ... " or "I'm confused ... " or "I'm irritated ... "

Stopping the use of questions needs to be done carefully to avoid rejecting the questioner. After her initial intervention, the teacher may need to focus on making members aware of the frame of reference of the questioner. Some are ready and willing to avoid asking questions in an effort to improve communication. Others are reluctant to do so, and further intervention may be required to gain their acceptance. A brief example of beginning intervention to avoid questions and encourage "I" statements is included here.

Sam: Why don't you feel like talking about this, John?
Teacher (intervention): "Sam, you haven't told John what your concerns are about this. I feel you would be more helpful to John, if you made it clear what you have in mind.
Sam: John, I guess I'm having difficulty relating to your reluctance to talk about this issue. I don't feel this way. I would like to talk about it and clear the air.

In this case, Sam makes an "I" statement and communicates more openly and clearly to John.

Gossip. Gossip also inhibits communication. Members are talking about another member rather than speaking directly to her, often while she is sitting in the midst of the conversation. The teacher intervenes and asks the member talking to speak directly to the other member concerned. For example:

Ann: I'm mad at Kim for not coming better prepared.

Sue: I agree with you, Ann. Kim is not contributing her share. She's not helping us very much.

Teacher (intervention): Sue, you are talking about Kim. Could you please try and speak directly with her?

Sue: Kim, I'm mad too. I wish you would work with us. We could get a lot more done.

By speaking directly to Kim, Sue is communicating in a much more direct fashion, rather than controlling Kim by ignoring her presence.

Super-mothering. Super-mothering occurs when people intervene in confrontations in an effort to alleviate hostility, guilt and pain. It inhibits communication. The intervention is usually a soothing, "smothering" comment. While the intensity of the confrontation is lessened and may be diverted, a member may be denied the opportunity to air some intra- or interpersonal conflict that might be a source of growth for her. The teacher intervenes to try to divert the super-mothering comment so that the confrontation can be completed to resolution. The following dialogue illustrates this behavior:

Mary: Jim, when you talk all the time, I get mad. I want a chance to talk, too.

Elaine (to Mary): Jim doesn't mean anything by it. He's got a lot of good information.

Teacher: Elaine, it seems to me you are denying Mary's feelings; she is saying something that she wants Jim to hear.

The teacher's intervention allows the conflict that Mary is feeling to be dealt with openly in a transaction with Jim. It stops Elaine from smoothing over the situation to hide the conflict and avoid the confrontation.

Speaking for someone else. Speaking for someone else is an inhibiting dynamic that occurs when one participant makes assumptions about what another is thinking or feeling. The member who is thus "interpreted" is negated as a person. There is a subtle difference between speaking for someone and offering feedback. In the former, a participant is reading another's thoughts, whereas in the latter, the participant delivering feedback is taking full responsibility for her thoughts and feelings. The teacher raises the students' awareness of this dynamic when it occurs. As illustration:

Heather: I'm sure I can speak for Barbara when I say that we are in complete agreement with . . . or:

Heather: Speaking for Barbara and myself, this situation is ridiculous! or:

Heather: It's obvious to me that this situation is frustrating to all of us.

Teacher (intervention): Heather, I'm not sure you can speak for anyone else but yourself. Otherwise, you may be attributing thoughts or feelings to people that may not necessarily be theirs. However, I'd like to hear from you.

The teacher encourages the student to speak for herself, in effect, saying that the student is important enough as a person to be heard. At the same time, she is preventing the student from controlling others by speaking for them. This says to the other members, "You, too, are important enough to be heard."

Invasion of privacy. Invasion of privacy may occur when members are allowed to question one another. The necessity for avoiding questions for other reasons has already been discussed. Those comments apply here also. The fact that questions threaten people and invade their privacy is another reason to avoid them.

As members of clinical nursing groups are adults, they can usually safely volunteer material from their own lives, and can exercise judgment as to what to bring into a group and what to avoid. The teacher, however, must always be alert to any content that could potentially hurt the group members or their families. She intervenes to block any discussion of personal content that could represent an invasion of privacy. She accomplishes this by focusing on concerns and feelings the members are experiencing, usually related to their current discussions and learning experiences. She does not allow any discussion of people and their problems if they are not present.

Marcia: Is it true that Debbie [another student] had a hypophysectomy to help her control her diabetes?

Teacher (to Marcia): Perhaps you could talk about your concerns for Debbie personally with her.

In this example, the teacher has not rejected the questioner, yet has effectively blocked any invasion of Debbie's privacy. Another illustration might be:

Marcia: My teenagers got into it last night. They had both been drinking.

Teacher: I feel a little uncomfortable right now listening to how fast you are talking, the feeling of anger in your voice and seeing your unhappy expression.

Marcia: Okay I guess I still feel uptight. I can't seem to unwind. I feel like yelling at everyone here or hitting someone.

In this situation, the teacher has turned the focus of Marcia's conversation from her children, who were not there, and centered it on helping Marcia become aware of what she is feeling. She helped Marcia to get in touch with her bodily reactions, and through them, with the feelings she was having. Ultimately, Marcia was even able to own these feelings and to express them in the group. Awareness is a first step in personal growth. Often it is necessary to intervene in situations like this to provide appropriate outlets for feelings so that they can be shared and dealt with openly. This allows the group to proceed effectively with its work, less inhibited by hidden agendas.

Processing the Progress of a Group. Feedback based on the teacher's perceptions is an important resource to be used by the group as a whole to correct its behavior and thereby better accomplish its goals. For example, a group of five students was discussing anatomy, physiology and pathophysiology in relation to specific cognitive objectives of a pharmacology assignment. The members, obviously having come prepared, were busy tossing out ideas and statements, however, no one was building anyone else's ideas. There was little supporting of each other, no attending skills with active listening or responding evident, chairs were spaced wide apart and no consensus or conclusions could be reached. Little progress was being made toward accomplishing the cognitive task. After joining the group and observing the difficulty it was having, the teacher confronted the group with its problem as she perceived it.

Teacher: It seems to me that you are experiencing some difficulty with working together and accomplishing the task today. (The group members were silent at first.)

Student A: I'm really tired and not very interested in the task.

Student B: I want to get on with it, but we don't seem to be getting anywhere.

Student C: No one is really interested or very talkative today. It was a lot of reading.

Teacher (nodding her head slightly): In other words, some of you are bored, others frustrated and discouraged? (General shaking of heads but no verbal replies.) I wonder if I could share with you for a few minutes some of the things that I see happening that might be contributing to the situation? (Group members nodded in agreement, some grinned nervously.)

Your chairs are wide apart, so much so, that it appears to be difficult for you to hear each other easily. When you are not speaking, you are not paying attention to the person who is talking. You are not even looking in her direction. Remember the importance of attending skills? I do not see many being used. Each one of you is coming prepared and offering pieces of information. This is good, however, I do not see you working together, building on each others' ideas to produce a whole pattern in which all the pieces come together. (Pause . . .) How does what I'm saying fit in with what you are experiencing? How does it feel to be talking and offering a good idea, when no one else cares to listen? (Silence from the group members. No eye contact with the instructor. She waits a few minutes and continues). I would like you to take a few minutes and talk with each other about what is happening to you right now—what is happening in the group—what your reactions are to the observations I shared with you—what you are learning from this experience.

The teacher left the group alone to discuss the feedback she had offered. As she observed the group from across the room, the students began to lean forward in their chairs and talk rapidly and earnestly. There was some laughter. Suddenly the members began pulling their chairs closer together. After ten minutes, the teacher returned for a brief period to check how the group was doing. She listened for a few minutes. The group had moved on from the affective task of discussing its behavior to working in earnest on the cognitive task. Near the end of the session, the teacher again joined the group and entered the discussion, pointing out the positive change in the group's behavior and its increase in productivity. She asked if the members would be willing to share with each other what they had learned from the experience.

Student D: I feel better. I kind of liked being able to talk about what was happening in our group. It seemed to help us. We began to help each other afterward.

Student E: It was hard, I was scared at first to say how I felt until I heard someone else say she was uncomfortable. Then I could say I was too.

Student A: I felt good being able to say that I didn't really know how to work in a group, that I prefer to work alone, but that I would try this and see what happened. No one said I was bad for feeling this way, and I felt closer to everyone after saying how I felt.

Student B: We were able to get on with our other work once we got unstuck, and we were so much better at it then.

Student C: I'm still not sure I want to do this all the time, but if I have to I will. I did get some questions answered that I wouldn't have if you had been here because I would have been afraid to ask them.

Teacher: Yes, it's nice to be able to turn to your peers and know you can depend on them to help you. I want to thank each of you for sharing. I heard one of you use the word unstuck. It seems to me to describe very aptly what happened in your group. Once you got yourselves unstuck, you accomplished a lot of work here today, and you seem to feel pretty good about this.

In her role as participant the teacher provided specific feedback from a positive orientation that the group was able to use in assessing its interactions, making some changes in its behavior and moving onward toward its goal. This kind of intervention locates responsibility for the running of the group and the accomplishment of the learning task, whether it be cognitive or affective, with the students. By doing this, the teacher is saying to the group members, "I have confidence in you, but I am here to help you when you need it." The teacher helped the group gain knowledge by looking at itself and it objectives. This becomes additional material that the group can use in moving more effectively to achieve future cognitive and affective goals. At the same time, members learn to get along with each other and to participate effectively in a group setting.

The participant role of leadership that best facilitates the ongoing processing of group behavior is one in which the teacher does not control or steer the group. Instead, in democratic fashion, she provides the group with ideas to be tested, critically evaluated and challenged. In the illustration, the teacher suggests that the group is having a problem, the members can agree or disagree. She suggests they look at their behavior and discuss it; the members can agree or disagree to do this. Most important, she does not control or manipulate them while they are discussing their behavior. Thus she demonstrates confidence in their ability to be responsible and accountable for directing and controlling their own behavior.

In conclusion, we see that the main activity of a participant teacher is to provide feedback to individuals or to the group about behavior and its effects. This is in line with the Gestalt assumption that if people can be more aware of their actions and the consequences of these actions, they can use this information to work more effectively. This assumption seems reasonable, but is no guarantee that sheer awareness will be effective in producing needed change. Yet without awareness and knowledge of behavior and its effects, there is little chance to adjust and improve either individual or group performance.

Feedback is the crux of the teacher's participant role in facilitating the growth of individuals and the group. The background that makes it possible to develop helpful feedback and deliver it is derived from the teacher's resources of knowledge about group process and effective communication.

Teacher as Resource

The teacher who uses group process as a teaching method basically serves as a resource for three major areas: (1) a content area of expertise (subject matter), (2) effective communication skills and (3) group process, its development and function. She is responsible, for the most part, for assigning learning tasks so that students can achieve objectives in an experiential manner from any one of these three areas. She assumes this responsibility because she has the broad picture of the final desired outcome, toward which all the individual learning objectives and tasks are aimed. Another term for her role might be that of coordinator of learning experiences.

The tasks that the teacher assigns the group may be either cognitive or affective in nature or, more likely, a combination of the two. A cognitive task often requires discussion of particular subject matter according to specific guidelines and objectives. An affective task can be to ask group members to share their current feelings and reactions or discuss how they are getting along together in achieving their goals. A combination task might be one that concerns a content area, but includes both cognitive and affective components. An example of this would be the following:

Content area: Provide nursing intervention for a female patient with cancer who has had a recent mastectomy and may be discharged soon.

Task: Students in small groups (four or five) will take turns role playing, with one student taking the part of a nurse and another student the part of the patient. The student playing the role of nurse will use appropriate attending and responding skills (affective component) when communicating with the patient. She will also select one content area (cognitive component) appropriate to meeting this patient's learning needs. This might be information about her forthcoming radiation and chemotherapy treatment, various recommended arm exercises, types and availability of breast prostheses or community resources accessible to help her when she is discharged.

When students are not actually involved in the role playing, they will be observers, concentrating on the type of communication present, the reactions of the nurse and the patient to each other and the appropriateness and accuracy of cognitive information conveyed to the patient by the nurse. At the end of one timed role playing situation (five minutes), the observers will give descriptive behavioral feedback on what they observed, i.e., attending and responding skills used, feelings and reactions expressed and completeness, pertinence and appropriateness of the cognitive information offered. About three minutes is allotted for completion of this task. Students then spend two minutes sharing their own feelings and reactions to the learning experience (personalized affective component). At the end of this, the exercise is repeated with the students assuming different roles.

This sample situation demonstrates the integration of the cognitive and affective realms of learning. The setting in which the learning activity occurs is a small group that provides each student with more opportunity to talk and share than she would have in a large group. The task itself promotes interaction and involvement among the students. The learning is student-centered. The teacher acts as a resource person and monitors the ongoing interactions of the group members and the functioning of the group, ready to intervene and provide feedback if she determines that it is needed. Students learn to participate as effective members of a group.

Perhaps it would be helpful to include a few words about the actual process of assigning any kind of task to a group. It has been our experience that an unclear task assignment interferes with the whole desired learning activity.

The task needs to be specific, concise and concrete with examples offered to clarify it, if need be. The assignment should be repeated slowly at least two times to ensure that all students hear what it is. If possible, a brief description can be written on the blackboard to allow the students to continue to refer to it as necessary.

Whenever feasible, it is helpful to give process instructions, i.e., talk students through the exercise step by step. For example, one could begin by saying,

"Next we will be working on attending skills. Let's all stand up." (Pause until everyone is standing.) Then, "Now select a partner and decide who will be A and who will be B." (Pause again, until action is completed.) Then, "Okay, A begin talking about something that you learned during your clinical experience that is important to you today. B, listen to A using the attending skills we discussed. Do not speak to A—only listen using attending skills." Giving instructions in this way prevents overloading of the information and maximizes the opportunities for students to raise questions to clarify confusion if it occurs. Answer all questions clearly and concisely throughout the exercise, and if there are any at its completion.

These suggestions will contribute toward the presentation of a clear task that will keep the group moving forward in its work. Members will not have to spend valuable time determining what a teacher meant by the assignment. There are some other points that will help to manage the learning activity smoothly:

Keep the exercise moving by keeping track of the time and announcing changes, or assign a group member to do this if you are unable to do it. Also, try to keep the pacing even so that each person spends equal time on an activity. Otherwise someone may feel short-changed.

Keep interaction periods as brief as possible—two minutes or less, usually. Again, this depends on the particular learning activity. You will need to be the judge of your timing. Some of our examples in Chapter 6 will include timing that has worked for us.

When moving from one activity to another, it is helpful to give a brief summary of what the group has been doing thus far and what they will be doing next. These points help students to retain an understanding of the broader perspective of the whole learning situation. Time should be set aside with each activity for students to share new insights and learning they have gained, as well as feelings and reactions to the experience.

Cognitive Content. Knowledge of subject matter should enable the teacher to serve as a resource person for cognitive information. She fulfills the responsibilities of this role differently as a manager of group process, however, than she would as a didactic presenter of cognitive information. She does not offer a prepared lecture of information she considers important for the students to learn. Instead, she plans for and arranges group activities that will assist the students in learning the appropriate content and skills she knows they must master to be competent. She helps the group and individuals to evaluate their growth in the cognitive area. A simple group quiz would be an illustration of this.

If a group or individual is having difficulty with grasping particular principles and understanding certain facts, she may do one of four things:

1. Offer explanations to clear up the misunderstandings of the subject matter.
2. Suggest alternative resources, articles, books and audiovisual materials that

provide different or simpler approach as to the information.

3. Help the students develop and use a problem-solving approach to determine the cause of their difficulty (it could be a simple lack of preparation on the part of group members, or problems with the functioning of the group).
4. Support individual and group decisions for corrective action that will help acquire the necessary cognitive learning.

As a resource person in the cognitive area, the teacher is responsible and accountable for determining and meeting the objectives for that area. She is the one who establishes what content must be learned. The instructor who uses a didactic approach in her teaching and the teacher who uses a group process approach have the same responsibilities for teaching cognitive content. The difference is that the teacher using group process needs additional resources in communication and group process. Expertise in these additional areas enables her to personalize and humanize her teaching.

Communication. In several ways the teacher is a resource person for the learning of effective communication skills. She provides feedback to increase student awareness of the kind of behavior that opens communication channels and the kind that closes them. This function needs active attention as the group begins its activities, and less so as the members learn group membership responsibility. She serves as a model of effective communication, and demonstrates constructive ways for offering feedback. She arranges activities in which students experience as well as practice effective communication skills, and makes available cognitive resource information about these skills.

The one area of communication that seems to warrant further exploration is helpful ways to give feedback. As we have seen, feedback is the crux of the teacher's role as a participant. In fact, it is a critical component of all communication. In group process, students are provided with multiple opportunities to practice giving feedback. In this, the teacher serves as a role model. Most of the characteristics of effective feedback were reviewed and illustrated earlier. The following is a synopsis of these characteristics. Helpful feedback is:

1. Specific rather than general.
2. Focused on behavior rather than on the person (what a person does rather than what she is).
3. Concerned about the needs of the person to whom it is directed (if it only serves the needs of the giver, it can be destructive).
4. Directed toward behavior about which the recipient can do something.
5. Most helpful when it has been actively solicited by the recipient.
6. A sharing of information rather than giving of advice.
7. Appropriately timed—immediate feedback is most useful, considering first the person's readiness to hear it, support systems available from others, and so on.

8. Restricted to the amount of information that can be used by a recipient so that it is not overwhelming.
9. Concerned about what is said or done, but not how or why.
10. Checked to see if the recipient understands it.

Another aspect of effective feedback is the way in which it is offered. For this, the use of effective communication skills is essential because they can build a climate of trust and confidence, mutual acceptance and support. In this kind of atmosphere, feedback can be appreciated as being a response given out of genuine concern, to help rather than to hurt. The skills that contribute to this atmosphere are briefly reviewed:

Attend to the person: This helps him feel you are interested and concerned about him and leads to a feeling of sharing and to the development of mutual concern. This behavior also tends to encourage an individual to refine his ideas and express himself more efficiently because he realizes others are listening to him.

Paraphrase what the other person has said before you give any feedback: This helps the speaker identify and focus on aspects of a situation that are contributing to his feelings. It encourages further exploration and examination of what was said.

Reflect the feelings of the person before you offer feedback: This raises that person's awareness to affective issues that he might otherwise not consider. It helps him to become aware of what his feelings are that lie behind the content of what is being discussed.

Reflect the behavior: This allows a person to see his behavior as it is observed by others, which adds a whole new dimension to his perspective.

Offer support: This encourages a person to feel secure enough to participate. It also helps him to feel less threatened.

Confront or challenge when appropriate: As feedback can provide confrontation or challenge, this encourages members to deal directly and more openly with each other. The goal of confrontation is to present a challenge, but to do so in a way that is helpful. Its purpose is to help a person stop and look at his behavior, of which he might otherwise have been unaware. (See Chapter 4 for a discussion of helpful forms of confrontation that need not be aggressive or hostile forms of communication.)

Summarize: This helps a group or individual to review past activities or reactions, and consider possible directions. It helps to establish an agenda for future sessions and highlights unresolved issues. An instructor can do the summarizing or can ask the group or an individual to do it for a particular time period.

Clarify: This helps to eliminate misunderstandings and distortions in communication. The teacher may simply ask a person to clarify what was meant by his remarks. This will help to avoid needless conflict.

Link: Linking together ideas and feelings, verbal and nonverbal messages or one member's comments with another's is often helpful, contributing to a feeling of unity.

The skills that contribute to creating acceptable feedback are important parts of communication as a whole, and are vital to the teacher who uses group process as a method of teaching.

Group Process. The teacher must have some working knowledge of how groups develop and function. Ultimately, she must integrate this knowledge with her background in the areas of cognitive content and communication skills.

When she has integrated all of this material into a unified approach, her most difficult problem is most likely to be that of timing—when to intervene and put her resources to work. Timing requires a careful and sensitive assessment of the instructor's observations. There are no hard and fast rules. Experience in using group process and practice in making interventions are probably the best teachers. A few points that have been helpful to us are:

1. Before you take risks and intervene with feedback, it is helpful if you first develop a trusting and supportive climate, in which the members feel secure with themselves and with you. Sometimes we find it helpful in the beginning stages of a new group to remove ourselves to allow time for the members to begin to establish relationships and build up trust and confidence in each other, without the presence of an authority figure.

2. Avoid waiting until near the end of a session to point out areas that need improvement. There may not be enough time left in the session to do this, and group members are left hanging without the time needed to do the work.

3. If it is late in the session, sometimes summarizing by the teacher or by the group may be helpful in looking at what the group has done and what it might do in the future.

4. If the group is just beginning work during a session, avoid intervening early unless they have been working together for several weeks or days.

5. Feedback is usually most effective if it is offered immediately on observing, taking into consideration other points mentioned above, of course.

Hopefully, some of these suggestions will offer a beginning guide to sensitive timing of your management of group process. The teacher with a broad resource background base in cognitive content, communication and group process is well prepared to personalize learning for each student. This becomes possible when she combines her expertise in these three areas into an integrated whole and employs a group process method.

USE OF CONFLUENT TECHNIQUES

An ability to manage various types of confluent techniques is vital to a learning environment that is diverse, challenging and personalized. Considering this, it is appropriate to review a definition and description of confluent techniques.

These are techniques that by design create a situation in which both affective and cognitive growth are fostered. Confluent techniques foster process.

Process is defined[15] as "a continuing development involving many changes." In the classroom, process refers to the development involving intellectual and emotional change and growth of both teacher and student.

Many books have been written suggesting various confluent techniques that can be adapted for use within an established curriculum. They are helpful, however, only if they become part of a whole confluent approach. If they are used only once in a while they have little value or meaning in achieving humanistic education. Confluent techniques are not used in our curriculum for "turn-on games" to excite people and provide something new and interesting momentarily, or for the effect of an individual technique alone. Instead, they are part of an ongoing process directed toward facilitating holistic learning in the classroom.

Group process, which has already been discussed, is the major confluent technique that we use. Others that have proven exceptionally helpful to us in conjunction with our use of group process are: information intermix, role playing, simulation and fishbowl. These add variety to the students' group experience and have become integrated into the process approach to our conferences. Each is used with a specific purpose in mind and contributes to part of the total confluent experience of the students.

Uses of Groups

Group process makes possible a great variety of approaches to learning. The size of the groups can be altered, and the tasks changed. Each alteration, especially in size, changes the dynamics of the learning situation. The selection of which size group to use usually depends on the task that is to be assigned, the amount of time available, the stage of group development, the cohesiveness of the group and the objectives of the learning experience.

Group sizes may vary from our usual two groups of five members each, to several smaller ones of two or three members (diads and triads), to larger ones of ten students. Once in a while during the semester, we may combine two clinical groups to make a group of twenty members when increased input would be helpful.

The use of diads allows increased communication and involvement by individual students, helping to build trust and decrease anxiety. A student who may be having difficulty talking in a group of five peers can often be observed deeply involved and participating actively with another student on a one-to-one basis. Rotating from partner to partner provides the opportunity for her to have this kind of experience with all the students in the group. Soon she builds up familiarity and trust with each of the group members as individuals and develops greater confidence in her own capabilities. Her anxiety decreases. Eventually, she begins to participate more frequently in her group of five peers. For a shy student, this is often an entirely new experience. What is even more exciting is that her participation has occurred as a natural evolution of her own growth, and not as the result of external demands placed on her by the teacher. She is self-directed and self-motivated.

The use of triads adds the role of observer to the one-to-one relationship. After observing the communication between students in a diad relationship, the third student who is the observer practices providing direct, descriptive feedback about its quality to the other students. This is usually quite a new experience for most students, and may cause some anxiety in the beginning.

Throughout the semester, our clinical group of ten students most often works in two groups of five students each. This situation is flexible. At the close of a particular session, the teacher may bring the students together to share what they have learned with the larger group. The teacher is the manager of the process through task assignment, determination of group size and her various roles as model, observer, participant and resource person. She determines when additional confluent techniques would be useful and initiates them.

Information Intermix

Information intermix is a confluent technique that is adapted from the article *Information Intermix: An Approach to Group Guidance* by Dave Capuzzi[6]. The article describes the intermix method in detail and suggests that it be used as an approach to group guidance. We have adapted the method to meet our content curriculum needs in pre-clinical or post-clinical conferences where it has worked successfully. The following is a description of intermix as we use it:

Topic: Teaching of Counseling or Nursing Content Through Experiential Approach of Information Intermix.

Objectives.
The students will:
1. Practice attending skills.
2. Practice listening for content.
3. Practice paraphrasing.
4. Select a concept from assigned reading and teach it to another group member.
5. Review pertinent information from previously assigned reading through intermix activity.
6. Identify and share feelings generated by this experience.
7. Be responsible for own individual and other group members' learning.
Organization.
Student assignment: From assigned reading, select a concept (an idea, prin-

ciple, quote, aspect or point) and write it on a 3 x 5 card and bring it with you to class. You will be sharing it with other students.

Procedure used during class:

1. Students divide into their usual support groups of four to five.

2. Five minutes is allowed for sharing in small groups concepts that students have chosen. It is helpful to notify the groups when each minute or so is up. This assists them in allotting time for each member.

3. When sharing time is finished, each student will select a partner, never someone from her own group. They will decide who is A or B and sit facing each other.

4. Students take turns switching roles. First, A will teach B for one minute about the concept that she (A) brought with her. At the end of one minute, notify students of the time so that B can teach her concept to A. Total time is two minutes for teaching in this dyad situation.

5. Students change partners and follow the same procedure with one change. This time, after teaching their own concept, they will, in addition, teach the one they learned from their partner in the preceding dyad. Time allotted is one and a half minutes per student in this dyad. If the time is too long, students will stray from the topic. The brief time period encourages practice in condensing and paraphrasing information.

6. Students follow this procedure in one or two more dyad relationships. Each time they teach their own concept plus any others they learned from previous partners, accumulating several concepts throughout the process.

7. Students return to original support groups and teach their accumulated information. Time allotted for this teaching is about ten minutes.

8. Students compare and assess their original information with the total information they have gained. Time allotted is three to five minutes.

9. Students share feelings, new learnings and reactions they had from this experience. Time allotted is five minutes.

Special Comments.

1. At the end of one occasion of intermix activity have students identify, within their support groups, the objectives they feel were achieved and then have the small groups share this within the larger group.

2. If a student comes unprepared to class, it is necessary to separate her from the process, because of the interference created by the negative feelings of members who are prepared toward those who are unprepared. This should not be done in a punitive way. Another activity, i.e., a dialogue of some kind between unprepared members, or time to do the reading assignment they did not have time to complete, is substituted. Students have not objected to this handling of the situation. They usually come prepared the next time.

3. The 3 x 5 cards are signed by the students and collected by the instructor. This helps the teacher to identify the individual learning levels of the students and to be aware of the material that was discussed.

4. Information intermix technique has been used many times, with multiple variations imposed on its basic formula. It is helpful for initial building of trust at the beginning of the semester when groups are new. It continues to provide variety and interest to learning activities throughout the semester.

5. The best setting is a room that has movable desks or chairs.

6. When the procedure is used for the first time, a general introduction describing the process can be helpful. "You are going to be participating in a learning activity that will hopefully be quite enjoyable. It will encourage you to be helpful to one another and will not embarrass you or put you 'on the spot' in any way. You are responsible for your own learning as well as for your classmates' learning during this activity. Try to assimilate and remember as many ideas as you can during the activity. Discussion time will be provided at the end to allow you opportunity to express any feeling you may have generated during the session. Please listen carefully to directions."

While information intermix has worked well in our post-clinical conference sessions, it has not been as successful when we attempted to introduce it into our larger lecture classes. This was probably because it was a single confluent technique introduced into one class in the midst of a didactic sequence of classes. It was also a new approach for many students. Only part of the lecture group of sixty students had previously experienced a confluent approach in clinical conference sessions and resistance was great. The results of these individual trials supported the concept that if the techniques are to be of value in fostering humanistic education, they need to be part of a total confluent approach.

Role Playing

Role playing is a versatile technique that is adaptable to many situations. It can involve transactions with two or more people, or with the fragmented parts of a single person. It can be part of a preplanned learning activity for a particular conference session, or it can be used spontaneously should a need for it arise during a group session. Frequently, it is combined with a simulation activity (described below).

Most often in our conference sessions, role playing has been used in the traditional fashion with transactions occurring between two or more people. Sometimes, for example, students practice their teaching skills in role-playing situations designed to simulate reality. Students select and prepare to teach specified information related to the cognitive objectives of the week and to their patient assigments, taking turns being the patient or the nurse. This practice increases student awareness of the need for teaching the patient and improves teaching skills and the ability to apply learning principles. It also heightens recognition of the need for using lay language in patient education.

Periodically, students role play a situation in order to solve a problem. Exploring the situation in this manner offers them new perspectives and understanding of the problem. At other times, reverse role playing brings insight and understanding to the feelings and thoughts of those students involved in a conflict situation that may have occurred clinically or during a group session. To illustrate, Student A, involved in a conflict, assumes the role of the person opposing her in the real situation. Another student, B, takes the role of Student A. They act out the situation. A slightly different approach would be to have the student who presents the conflict, play both parts of the situation. Following each of these examples, students discuss and share their feelings. This helps them to gain insight and understanding of themselves and others.

While role playing other people has the advantages discussed, it is even more valuable to have students play themselves in diad, triad and small group interactions. Students have the opportunity realistically to practice their communication skills, to give and receive feedback and to improve areas that need strengthening as they become aware of them.

Because role playing can be used in many ways, it provides creative opportunities for experiential learning of new perspectives and insights and dynamics of situations that might not otherwise be possible.

Simulation

Simulation has been familiar in nursing education for a long time. The nursing arts laboratory for practicing bed-making and procedures is a well known example. Simulation is defined by Lincoln, Layton and Holdman[20, p. 316] as "a representation of reality for a specific purpose." There are multiple forms of simulation, some complex, others simple, each with varying degrees of comprehensiveness and reality.

The more complex a simulation is, the more comprehensive and representative it is of a broad range of reality. A simple simulation is less complex and comprehensive. The authenticity of a simulation also contributes to its complexity. The success of a simulation depends on whether or not it helps students fulfill the learning objectives of a particular situation.

Simulation techniques offer several advantages[9]. First, students enjoy participating in them. Second, they can involve several types of learning—cognitive, affective and psychomotor—in one learning event. Third, simulation activities can increase students' understanding of themselves and others. Fourth, they provide experiential learning, and this kind of learning seems to stay with the student longer. Fifth, the anxiety level of the students can be less, as they are not afraid of harming a real patient. Sixth, a highly sophisticated simulation can standardize the learning environment.

In our clinical conferences, we use a number of different simulation techniques, most of them simple to design but directly related to our curriculum. The more we use simulations, the easier they are to develop. Sometimes, they are preplanned. At other times, they are developed spontaneously to fulfill a need. They may demand performance of psychomotor, teaching, counseling or problem-solving skills. As an example, when students are studying sensory deprivation, they take blind-trust walks with partners, taking turns being the person who is blind. A similar activity is one in which students live with a simulated handicap for 24 to 48 hours. At the end of each of these activities, students share what the experience was like for them and what they learned from it. From these activities comes new awareness for students about how it feels to have a handicap and how they might better assist a patient who has one. Thus simulation is an effective confluent technique for teaching empathy, for practice in applying principles and concepts and for increasing self-understanding.

Fishbowl

The fishbowl technique is effective and fun to use. It can be used to teach feedback techniques, communication skills, group membership roles or problem solving. We have used it successfully to familiarize students with the various roles they can play as members of a group.

A smaller group of students sits within a larger group that acts as observers. The students in the center discuss a problem, usually assigned by the teacher. The students in the outside circle record how those in the inner circle helped or hindered group functioning. They indicate on a chart how students in the inner circle are performing the various functions of group members. Each student observer has her own chart.

The chart organizes the functions of group members into two major areas: helping functions and hindering functions. It includes definitions of these areas. The helping functions are further divided into two subgroups: task functions, which are related to achievement of the group task, and maintenance functions, which are concerned with developing and maintaining the proper emotional/social climate[4].

Helping Functions.

Task functions involve:

Initiating: Proposing and defining the task for the group.

Seeking information or opinions: Asking questions about relevant information, or asking for expression of feelings or personal value.

Giving information or opinions: Offering relevant information; stating opinions or expressing personal values.

Summarizing: Bringing ideas together so that the group can refocus on the problem; offering a conclusion that the group can accept or reject.

Clarifying: Clearing up misunderstanding and defining terminology; rephrasing a statement to facilitate understanding.

Consensus testing: Checking with the group to see whether they are reaching a decision.

Maintenance (emotional and social) functions include:

Encouraging: Supporting other group members; indicating through nonverbal gestures acceptance of another's thoughts.

Harmonizing: Trying to reconcile disagreements or to reduce the anxiety level.

Compromising: Agreeing to yield status or admit error so that the group can function.

Gate-keeping: Keeping channels of communication open; asking others to participate; suggesting procedures that allow others to participate.

Standard-setting: Exploring whether group members are satisfied with procedures.

Hindering Functions

Hindering functions include:

Seeking recognition: Calling attention to oneself through unusual behavior such as telling stories, boasting and loud talking.

Digressing: Getting away from the topic or the group task.

Out of field: Withdrawing from the discussion.

Blocking: Interfering with the group task by arguing excessively or by continually bringing up a "dead" issue.

In addition to these definitions, the chart that the student observers are using includes a check-off grid sheet on which to record the performances of the inner circle students as they take various roles (Figure 5-1).

Following the discussion by the students in the inner group, those students also receive copies of the same function charts. This helps them in developing awareness of the roles they were assuming. After a brief review, the students in the outer group give their feedback to the inner group. Based on the functions, they identify and describe the behavior they observed during the interactions of the inner group. The groups discuss this feedback. Eventually, both groups have an opportunity to describe their reactions to the experience and share what they learned from it.

FACILITATION OF GROUP DEVELOPMENT

The teacher sets the tone for the students response to group process. Her positive attitude as she explains to the students how it works is vital, as this frequently is their first exposure to this type of learning. Typically, our students react with confusion, curiosity or disbelief.

The first task for the teacher is to alter her behavior in order that she may serve as a role model for the type of behavior she expects of the students. The next task involves conducting specific learning activities that foster desired changes in the students' behavior. As stated earlier, our goal in post-clinical conference is to facilitate cognitive and affective growth through experiential learning. It is imperative that we design learning activities that bring about

---

Figure 5-1. Grid sheet for use in the fishbowl exercise.

Helping Roles

Student names

Task functions

1. Initiating						
2. Seeking information						
3. Giving information						
4. Summarizing						
5. Clarifying						
6. Consensus testing						

Student names

Maintenance (social and emotional) functions

1. Encouraging						
2. Harmonizing						
3. Compromising						
4. Gate-keeping						
5. Standard-setting						

Hindering Roles   Student names

Hindering functions

1. Seeking recognition						
2. Digressing						
3. Out of field						
4. Blocking						

changes in our students' knowledge, attitudes and skills. The activities must also use nursing content and reflect specific nursing goals so that the student can identify the relationship between group activity and desired outcomes.

In Chapter 4, we discussed the five stages of group development and examined the tasks the group must accomplish in each stage. The teacher's role is that of facilitator, as she creates an environment conducive to group process. She conducts group learning activities that provide the opportunity for behavioral change in order that a particular stage can be mastered. She also serves as a model of the desired behavior necessary to pass successfully through each stage.

It is helpful to review briefly the task of each stage in order to present some suggestions regarding modified classroom techniques, learning activities and teacher behavior. We would also like to share with the reader some specific learning activities we have used.

Stage 1: Orientation

In the orientation stage the major consideration for the teacher is to provide the student with necessary information. The student must know course requirements, objectives and goals, teacher expectations and instructional methods, as well as something about her fellow students.

We have found it helpful to spend our first pre-clinical and post-clinical conferences of the semester orienting students to the clinical facility and its function. This is usually done in one large group (approximately twenty students and two instructors) in order that all students may benefit from any questions asked. At this time, we also review clinical course requirements and evaluation criteria. All questions must be answered immediately and satisfactorily if anxiety is to be reduced. Areas that are crucial to the students (i.e., the nursing care plan format) may have to be repeated, as anxiety tends to block reception of messages.

After this general orientation, we separate into groups. Each instructor has ten students and works with two groups of five students. At this time it is helpful to spend some time getting to know each other. One way to facilitate this is to have each person, beginning with the instructor, introduce herself. This is usually an informative but non-threatening exercise. The instructor sets the tone. We usually tell the group how long we have been teaching nursing, where we went to nursing school or college and a bit about our family, hobbies, and so on. Frequently, students will ask why we went into nursing, and why we chose the area of nursing education. It is important to answer these questions in order for the student to relate to the person the teacher is, not to just a position. The teacher participates in this exercise as a role model of behavior facilitative to beginning to learn about other people. It is also important to create an environment conducive to equality, inclusion and sharing, which is enhanced by the arrangement of the chairs in a closed circle.

The next activity is the introduction of group process as a learning method. A simple explanation of the humanistic theory with emphasis on self-determination, self-actualization, experiential learning and responsibility for learning helps define its objectives. We tell the students our belief that "the most important person to an individual's learning is the individual, second in importance is the individual's peers, third is the library and fourth, maybe, is the teacher"[18, p. 22]. This usually draws mixed reactions, as our students are basically accustomed to more traditional teaching methods and have difficulty accepting their own value in their learning experience. Our basic premise is that each student is responsible for her own learning and that she will function as part of a group, assuming the added responsibility of contributing to the learning needs of other group members.

It is difficult to explain the mechanics of group process to students, since this method espouses experiential learning. Thus it is more comprehensible if the students are allowed to experience what the instructor has described. With this in mind, we put the students in a group process situation early in the orientation stage. Usually on the second clinical day the students are assigned at random to one of two small groups that are situated some distance apart from each other. Each group is given a fairly basic task, usually, to decide when and how they would like to receive their weekly clinical patient assignments, with a choice among several options. The students are asked to share their opinions in their small group and reach a consensus.

At this point the teacher has already served as a role model for sharing in the get acquainted exercise, she has provided the necessary instruction and directives for the group task and has established the groups. Frequently, a group has difficulty commencing the initial task and literally waits for the teacher to lead them. Just as frequently, the teacher has difficulty not stepping in and leading the group. We have found it helpful to remove ourselves from the environment, for five to ten minutes, either to a far end of the room or out of the room entirely. It takes some time in group development until the group is secure enough for the instructor to participate as a group member and not be a disruptive force or a group-acknowledged leader.

At the end of the allotted time, the students are asked to share their decision regarding the assigned task and also how they arrived at it. This helps them clarify the process employed by the group and begin to develop initial awareness of group process function. This activity also encourages some sharing of feelings in a concrete, non-threatening circumstance.

It is helpful at this point to ask the students how they felt about making a decision relevant to themselves, in a group, deriving consensus from shared opinions. We point out that the activity they have just completed is group process in action. While this is in actuality very rudimentary group process, most students react favorably to the extent of their involvement in decision making and the ease of sharing an opinion. It is important that the first experience with group process be as positive and non-threatening as possible. The teacher cannot expect students to be able to share personal feelings during the orientation stage, as they are still exploring the novelty of the situation and usually are somewhat mistrustful and cautious.

Another exercise that is appropriate to the orientation stage involves working with diads. This introduces another confluent technique and exposes students to sharing on a one-to-one basis. We usually ask each student to select a partner. For about three to four minutes they discuss changes they made in patient care on the second clinical day as compared to the first clinical day. One-to-one sharing is usually comfortable and the non-threatening, common discussion-matter facilitates active sharing and helps the students get to know each other better. With slight modification, this exercise might be used further to facilitate building trust in the students. This helps answer their concern as to how they will be treated in the group. Trust begins to develop as the student is allowed to see how the group reacts to her. In the diad, the task is increased by one more directive, "Tell how you *felt* about this change in your care plan." This introduces the sharing of personal feelings related to the student's own behavior, and affords her the opportunity to observe how a peer reacts to this disclosure.

We have observed resistant behavior in many forms during the orientation stage, regardless of how well planned and presented the task assignment was. In Chapter 6, we will deal with specific student responses, both positive and negative, to selected group process activities. Let it suffice here to say that group development in the orientation stage is usually uneven, sometimes downright bumpy. It is not unusual occasionally to have to confront resistance, review the objectives of the group process learning method and allow the students an opportunity to ventilate their feelings. Such ventilating sessions are in themselves a form of learning through group process.

Thus the teachers role during this stage of group development is one of modeling desired behavior and encouraging and supporting interaction that assists the students with adjustment to a new circumstance, a new environment and a new peer group. The teacher must also be a careful observer. Disruptive or distracting behavior may indicate that the orientation stage is moving ahead too quickly and becoming threatening. In this case, the topic or structure must be altered and made less threatening[26].

Before passing out of the orientation stage, the teacher must assess student readiness for Stage 2. The students should feel relatively comfortable with each other and a sense of trust should start to emerge. We have found it difficult to pinpoint passage from one stage to another, as the groups tend to ease in and out of stages, although it is usually quite easy to identify the group that has not mastered the orientation stage, as mistrust and superficial communication impede productivity. The number of orientation sessions necessary varies, and assessment by the teacher is necessary to determine the requirements.

Stage 2: Establishing Norms

The goal of Stage 2 is for the group to take responsibility for itself and learn to function in an independent, self-directing manner. "Two ingredients are necessary if the group is to take responsibility for itself: opportunities to learn the skills needed, and opportunities for the group to practice directing its own activities"[26, p. 78]. It is the teacher's responsibility to see that these opportunities are provided to the students through the planning and implementation of group process exercises.

It is difficult for all parties involved to shift to group-centered learning, but the teacher can provide practice in the skills necessary to assume this responsibility. As mentioned in Chapter 4, the group developmental tasks in Stage 2 include: group responsibility, responsiveness to others, interdependence (cooperation), decision making through consensus, and confronting problems. Several forms of teacher behavior can be employed during this stage. These include: random selection of group members, determining appropriate group size, a seating arrangement conducive to communication, explicit definition of task assignments, readiness to serve as an observer, participant and resource person and ability to serve as a role model for the desired behavior expected of the students.

Group Responsibility. Our first concern in Stage 2 is to establish group responsibility. Early in the semester, we begin to use our Friday morning pre-clinical conference as a pharmacology group process session. All students receive a pharmacology reading assignment that correlates with the week's subject content. They are asked to come prepared to discuss the assigned drugs with their group. Three or four general discussion questions are put on the blackboard to help guide discussion should the group choose to use them. At the end of the pre-clinical conference, one copy of a short multiple choice quiz is given out, and each group is directed to answer the questions based on consensus.

Many aspects of the norm establishment phase are incorporated in this activity. Each student is responsible for her own preparedness and for sharing her knowledge with the group. As learning pharmacology is the desired goal, appropriate listening skills are required. The first several pharmacology group sessions often flounder in organization, as the students are in the process of sharpening the skills necessary to carry out group process learning. In order to handle the drug quiz, the group must be able to cooperate, communicate and reach a decision by consensus. We have found this method to be an extremely successful way to integrate pharmacology into our curriculum. Furthermore, student evaluations at the end of the semester have consistently reinforced how much the students like this approach to learning pharmacology.

It is best for the teacher to avoid direct intervention in early sessions and allow the group opportunity to establish its own operative norms. It is important, however, that the teacher assist the members to evaluate their functioning as a group at the end of the conference time. This may be accomplished by going over the quiz answers. We usually bring our two small groups together when reviewing the quiz, in order to share answers and to clarify misinformation. The quiz is a part of the group exercise and is not graded. We usually ask each group separately to discuss how it might have functioned more effectively, and what the group might have done to help its members learn pharmacology better. Honest assessment of functional weaknesses is mandatory for group development so that the group members may modify their activity and improve their functioning.

We find these pharmacology conferences serve as a helpful tool for the teacher in evaluating group development, as the general task assignment is consistent and the conferences continue every Friday all semester. It is interesting to note how much more informative, effective and efficient these conferences become throughout the semester as the students develop mastery of group process skills.

Another exercise that fosters group responsibility, cooperation (interdependence) and consensus is the "Mystery Diagnosis" exercise mentioned in Chapter 4. Several signs, symptoms or laboratory test results are written on 3 x 5 cards, one to a card. The cards are distributed among the group members, and they must pool their information and arrive at an agreed on diagnosis. The group is then asked to formulate an appropriate nursing care plan. At the end of the post-clinical conference the two groups compare their "mystery diagnosis" and share their nursing care plans. Then the groups are asked to discuss among themselves difficulties they may have experienced with the assignment and ways they might have solved the mystery more expediently.

We find it helpful for the teacher to withdraw during the groups' initial organizational attempts in each exercise and then casually to observe their process while circulating between them. This makes the instructor available for questions or clarification, but not available as a controlling or manipulating leader, and hopefully not as a distraction.

Responsiveness to Others. The students soon realize that task accomplishment is impossible unless all members contribute. Similarly, they find productivity comes to an absolute standstill if all members talk at once or interrupt each other. Inevitably, one or both of these situations do occur. The teacher usually recognizes this problem before the students do. When this occurs, it is helpful to incorporate some attending and responding exercises into the post-clinical conference to improve listening skills and motivate the students' responsiveness to each other.

Exercises that are helpful to develop responsiveness to others and good listening skills involve the use of diads and triads. Initially, after explaining the aforementioned desired outcomes of the exercise, we review the principles of active listening with the students, including: looking directly at the speaker, nodding to indicate attentiveness, paraphrasing pertinent information and identifying content and feeling. We set up diads and assign one person the role of speaker, and the other the role of listener. The speaker talks for two minutes about a patient problem she identified, the nursing intervention employed to meet the problem, and the rationale behind the intervention. The listener then paraphrases in thirty seconds the content presented by the speaker. Then both members discuss the outcome of the exercise. The speaker discusses whether she:

1. Felt that she was being listened to.
2. Felt encouraged to continue speaking.
3. Was distracted or discouraged by the listener.
4. Got her content across to the listener.

The listener is asked to discuss:

1. Problems she encountered with listening.
2. Things the speaker did that were distracting.
3. Difficulties she encountered in keeping the speaker talking.
4. Her ability to receive content messages from the speaker.

The students then switch roles and repeat the exercise.

A variation involves the use of triads, with one student assuming the role of the speaker, one the listener and one the observer. The speaker is asked to speak on something that has personal meaning, positive or negative, and related to nursing. The listener is to practice active listening, then respond by paraphrasing content and identifying the speaker's feeling regarding the content. The observer reports her observations of the speaker's ability to get her content across, and the listener's helpful and non-helpful attending behavior, accurate identification of feeling and recall of content. The same group rotates two more times so that each student has an opportunity to assume each role. At the end of the exercise, the students go back into their small groups and discuss what they learned about positive and negative attending and responding skills, and how this might be applied to both their group and patient interactions. A major force in teaching listening skills is the teacher's ability to practice them.

Interdependence. We have found establishment of cooperation as a group norm a relatively easy task. Our post-clinical conferences are not graded, so competition is eliminated as an obstacle to cooperation. Most of our students have a natural impulse to help each other, and this impulse is fostered by group process. We have found it helpful to have students practice basic principles of teaching and demonstrate their application in student one-to-one teaching situations. This assists the students in their efforts to help each other, and in their efforts toward patient education.

There are many exercises the teacher might use to foster cooperation. When teaching cardiopulmonary resuscitation (CPR), we assign two teams of two students each to a mannequin. The first team performs two-man rescue CPR, while the second team observes and makes helpful suggestions. Eventually, all four students rotate so that each student has practiced CPR with the other three and has served as an observer with each of the others.

An exercise to improve intragroup cooperation involves assigning each student a specific congenital cardiac anomaly to present and discuss with the group. After all five students have made their presentations and answered any questions, the group is given a packet of diagrams of all five anomalies. The diagrams have been cut into puzzle pieces and mixed up. The task assignment is for the group members to find the pieces of puzzle needed to construct the diagram of their assigned anomaly. They must do this without speaking to each other, motioning or pointing. They may not take a piece from another member, but must wait until it is passed to them. They may pass any of their puzzle pieces to any other member at any time. The two five-member groups usually view this exercise as an intergroup competition, which tends to increase their intragroup cooperation.

Decision Making through Consensus. As the groups' cooperation skills increase, their ability to reach consensus decisions improves. The caring attitude of cooperation fosters a sense of fairness and a willingness to listen to individual input. The teacher can help facilitate this developmental task by using consensus technique in all shared decisions. The teacher should always avoid show-of-hands majority rule, and encourage each student individually to offer her opinion and rationale relevant to the decision to be made. This emphasizes the equality the teacher places on each student and reinforces the student's sense of value and worth.

Confronting Problems. The final consideration of Stage 2 is that of problem confrontation. Few people are comfortable with direct confrontation of a problem. The natural human tendency when faced with an interpersonal problem is to avoid confrontation and hope the problem will go away. It usually does not. Nothing can be resolved unless it is confronted, and it is well to remember that even confrontation does not guarantee resolution. It is important for the teacher to explain to her students that for problems to arise within a dynamic interactive group is normal. The students should be helped to view problem confrontation as a growing, learning experience. "Confronting interpersonal problems openly is essential if a group is to develop its maximum effectiveness[26, p. 204].

There are many ways in which the teacher may be helpful in teaching students how to confront interpersonal problems. Initially, as an observer, the teacher usually recognizes the existence of a problem and the behavior that is causing it before the students involved do. The teacher's feedback of her observations brings the problem to the group's attention and provides an opportunity for them to deal with it.

We have found it helpful to allow the group the chance to define their problem behavior themselves, as they see it. Frequently an approach such as, "How well were your learning needs met in post-clinical conference today?" will initiate a discussion revealing the students' awareness of impeding behavior within the group. If they rather than the teacher identify and describe the behavior causing the problem, it will probably be dealt with more openly and honestly.

In problem confrontation the teacher should emphasize that the students must describe specific behavior and not speak in generalities. They must not try to second-guess what someone else is thinking, e.g., "Joan really doesn't seem to care about the group's work." Rather, they must describe exactly what behavior they feel is negative, e.g., "Joan, you have come without notes to conference on three occasions and did not contribute to group discussion on those days." Specific descriptions of observed behavior help the student to avoid being judgmental. The other members of the group should be asked if they have observed this behavior also, and each should be encouraged to describe whatever group behavior she feels is contributing to the problem.

We found it helpful to use group evaluation forms at least twice a semester, usually at the half-way point and at the end. The form (adapted from Stanford[27, pp. 121, 123]) asks the following questions:

1. Do you have a chance to talk as much as you want to in group?
2. Are you happy during the discussions? If not, why not?
3. What could members of the group do to make you more satisfied during discussions?
4. Does one person do most of the work of the group?
5. When you speak does everyone listen? If not, why not?
6. Does everyone contribute toward the work of the group?
7. What attempts are being made to include all members?
8. Does anything "bug" you during the discussions? If so, what?
9. How effectively is the group working toward its goals?
10. What problems does it seem to be having?
11. What should the group do to improve its functioning?
12. Do you like group process as a form of post-clinical conference?

The students fill out the evaluation questionnaire individually and then discuss each question in the group. We have used this form or a shorter modification on occasions when a group was having serious problems, to help them identify the source of the problems and to serve as a springboard for discussion.

Our students have been very responsive to the group evaluation, especially after receiving assurances that problems are normal and can be confronted in a constructive manner. We often observe the discussion dealing with problem confrontation to see that the students do approach the problem from a behavioral and not a personality standpoint. We have found most of our students to be honest and kind in these evaluations and usually able to pinpoint the impeding behavior quite clearly and accurately. In their evaluation discussion, the students usually include suggestions that they feel might resolve the problem. This type of problem confrontation skill fosters the group's responsibility to monitor its own behavior and is infinitely more effective than an authoritarian "scolding" from the teacher.

Stage 3: Coping with Conflict

When a group has developed cohesiveness and a comfortable feeling with each other, the members feel free to express their opinions and feelings, and also to disagree with each other. In the norm development stage, they learned how to confront problems that arise from conflicts perhaps as simple as a difference of opinion. Confrontation is a healthy developmental aspect of group process, but the very act of confrontation creates an open expression of conflict. Once students learn that intragroup problems must be confronted to be resolved, they need to learn the skills necessary to cope with the resultant conflict.

Conflict itself is not inherently bad. It frequently results in new ideas and methods that foster personal growth. What can be bad is the manner in which people respond to conflict. Therefore it is important for the teacher to stress positive aspects and reassure the students that it can be properly handled without being destructive and sacrificing someone's self-esteem.

The teacher can be helpful in guiding the students through coping with conflict by emphasizing the importance of active listening. They must learn to hear the content and feeling underlying the speaker's words. For example, "You say everything's all right, but you sound angry with me. What is making you angry?" Responding to a student's words and feelings acknowledges both and demonstrates acceptance of them. This acknowledgment and acceptance is the first step toward dealing with the underlying causes of the conflict. Exercises in attending and responding skills, described earlier, are of real help.

One of the outstanding problems in coping with conflict is placing guilt for the conflict on another person. Typically we hear, "You make me so angry," "Well, that was your own fault," "You really are thoughtless," "You just don't seem to care." This approach immediately puts the listener on the defensive. As she assembles and initiates her defensive response, conflict heightens rather than resolves.

The above examples are "you" messages—"you make me feel. . . ." They are usually destructive and negative. Stanford[26] recommends an exercise involving sending "I" messages. The students are asked to practice these messages in diad role playing. The situation involves a specific patient-nurse interaction that may be fictional or real. The person role playing the nurse must begin every response with "I"—"I sense you feel . . .," "I feel . . .," "I hear you say. . . ." As the students become more skilled at sending "I" messages, they may be encouraged to use this approach in coping with conflict within the group. The following steps should be included:

1. Identification of the problem (in behavioral terms) that is causing the conflict.
2. Description of the student's own feelings regarding the problem using "I" messages.
3. Use of active listening during each student's input, with paraphrased feedback of content and identification of feelings.
4. Contributions of possible alternatives to resolve the problem.
5. Negotiation of a solution derived by exploring the members' feelings regarding each alternative, and arriving at a consensus decision.

It is important that the final solution be agreeable to all if the group is to expect honest commitment to the solution.

The teacher can review and demonstrate each step in the coping process and then assign a task conflict for the group to resolve using the process. A basic task, such as "nursing students should/should not be required to hand in mini-care plans on a weekly basis," affords the students an opportunity to practice conflict coping skills and, hopefully, to develop some confidence in the process as a workable solution to dealing with conflict in their personal and professional lives.

Another helpful exercise is role reversal. We have used this with students who have had difficulty in interpersonal relationships with patients. The student who experienced difficulty with a patient plays the patient's part, and a second student plays the student's part. It has been interesting to note how much insight the student playing the patient gains into the motivations behind her patient's behavior. She develops a more objective perspective of her patient's point of view by playing his role. The one playing the student role has not been emotionally involved in the actual conflict situation and thus is often able to deal with the patient in an innovative, objective manner. Other students in the group may be asked to assume one or both roles, and role play the same conflict situation, affording still another perspective for coping with the problem.

These types of exercises demonstrate positive, constructive, relatively comfortable ways to deal with conflict. As conflict is an ever-present phenomenon in our personal and professional lives, learning to handle it effectively results in a higher level of personal development and growth.

Stage 4: Productivity

The productivity stage is a major milestone in group process development. The group has achieved the skills necessary for dynamic interaction and has become a mature, productive working unit. The members have learned how to deal with learning tasks efficiently and effectively. They have developed their communication skills to the point where they can deal constructively and comfortably with differing opinions and interpersonal conflict.

During this stage, group activity is divided between task functions and interpersonal functions, both of which are important parts of education. There is an increased intimacy between the students and toward the teacher that is constructive in that it fosters a sense of working together for the enrichment of all.

It is not uncommon, however, for problems to crop up during the productivity stage, although they are usually handled with ease. Regression occasionally occurs, manifested by withdrawal, disorganization or conflict. Many causative factors may enter into this. Typically, a vacation period such as spring semester break will cause a group temporarily to regress to an earlier behavior. Sometimes regression indicates a need for some review exercises in attending skills, or perhaps there is a problem within the group that has not been adequately confronted.

Sometimes a group becomes so close that all of its energies are spent on interpersonal functions. This, of course, diminishes productivity. Asking the group to evaluate its task assignment productivity following a clinical conference session often helps them realize they are not being as productive as they might be. When this decline in productivity is identified, it is helpful for the teacher to encourage the group to review its behavior during the conference. Members might be asked to identify which behaviors were task-oriented and which were social-oriented, and then determine the ratio. If too much time is being spent on building interpersonal relationships, the reason for reduced productivity should be clear.

We have found it quite rewarding to take advantage of the smooth, skilled group functioning in this stage to use some more highly developed group techniques. Two techniques that we have found to be very effective are role playing and simulation.

Role playing is one of the most effective methods of learning. We have found it especially helpful to have the students role play significant nurse-patient interactions (e.g., interacting with the terminal patient, or meeting specific patient teaching needs). Role playing affords the student a chance to practice her social and communication skills and to apply her cognitive background in a given situation. It also allows for freedom and flexibility on the student's part. Role playing is an excellent way to learn the effect of one's behavior and responses on others, as the interaction may be stopped at any point, with one or both role players asked, "How do you *feel* about what was just said?"

Effective role playing requires a well-developed group. Students can gain much insight by acting out a situation, but a student's ability to role play effectively will depend greatly on how secure and comfortable she feels with her fellow group members. A poorly developed group seldom benefits from role playing. Group members feel "silly" playing a role–they don't allow themselves to identify with the role or they give pat, stilted role responses. If a group has truly reached the productivity stage, they usually can handle role playing and find it an enjoyable, enlightening experience. (Specific examples of role playing situations are presented in Chapter 6.)

Simulation is another learning method that helps students to gain insight into how a person might think, feel and behave in a given situation. We employ several simulation exercises with our groups. One of the more popular and more difficult ones is used during our unit on disaster nursing. The students are given a simulated disaster and asked to list their behavioral responses in priority order, giving a rationale for each action and for its priority. The group carries out this task assignment together using consensus decision making. During the last ten minutes of conference, we ask the two groups to write their priority action lists on the board for comparison and discussion. For this simulation exercise, we have used the following format:

Disaster Simulation Exercise

Situation: You are an elementary school nurse. You have accompanied a teacher and 16 children, ranging in age from 6 to 11 years, on a school bus trip. On the return ride home, in a rather isolated area, the bus is involved in an accident with two cars. The post-accident status is as follows:

1. The bus has overturned and is lying on its side.
   a. The bus driver was thrown through the windshield and is unconscious on the pavement.
   b. Three children appear to be unresponsive.
   c. One child has an arm laceration that is spurting blood.
   d. Most of the children have multiple lacerations, and some demonstrate limb immobility.
   e. The teacher has glass fragments in her eyes.
   f. Several of the children are hysterical, some appear dazed.
2. Car #1
   a. Two occupants: a man and a woman.
   b. The woman is eight months pregnant and experiencing early labor pains; she appears relatively uninjured but is somewhat hysterical.
   c. The man is responsive. He is pinned behind the wheel and is having some difficulty breathing.
3. Car #2
   a. Car is flipped on its roof.
   b. One male occupant is trapped inside and is unresponsive.

Group Task Assignment: You, the school nurse, are uninjured. The only medical supplies are those found in the bus first-aid kit. Discuss your nursing priorities in this situation, and the rationale behind them. List each nursing intervention you would take in priority order and discuss the rationale behind the intervention and the priority rating.

This assignment demands considerable decision making concerning nursing assessment on both the physical and emotional level, principles of triage and functions of leadership role responsibility. The students really grapple with their nursing priorities and their discussion is usually very dynamic, focusing on the physical needs as well as the emotional needs of the injured. It is of interest to note that both groups of one of the teachers who used this exercise recently came up with identical priority listings.

Role playing and simulation are total involvement exercises. Both methods are very effective and both require a high degree of group interaction and maturity, and should not be undertaken extensively until a group has reached the productivity stage in its development.

Stage 5: Termination

This stage in group development is inevitable. The group members know from the start that ultimately the semester will end and their group will terminate.

A poorly developed group usually does not have strong feelings regarding termination, except, perhaps, relief that it is all over. A group that has progressed steadily through the developmental stages, however, usually has mixed feelings regarding termination. Typically, our students demonstrate a happy/sad type of behavior. They seem happy with the completion of their educational goal, yet, they appear sad, as if they are leaving something behind with which they really do not want to part. We find group task productivity starts to decrease in the last two weeks or so of the semester. The warm-up period is rather extended, and students tend to stray off topic more often as interest lags and apathy sets in. Conflict occasionally appears during this stage, and often the group has difficulty mobilizing their communication skills in order to deal with it productively. It is not uncommon for anger to be directed toward the teacher. This type of negative behavior indicates the students are having difficulty dealing with their mixed emotions regarding group termination.

The teacher can help the students realize and express their feelings and review the positive things they have learned from group process. Stanford[26, p. 268] says, "A 'good' termination helps students become aware of and express their genuine feelings, tie up loose ends, and resolve to reinvest their emotional energy in future experiences."

We use several exercises to help our students deal with termination. One involves the use of the group evaluation forms discussed on page 130. The members are asked to fill out the forms individually and then share their answers and feelings with the entire group. These evaluation forms usually yield positive comments and help the students see what they have accomplished and how the group has developed.

Another exercise involves listing on the blackboard as many of the semester's post-clinical conference activities as the group members can recall. They then discuss (1) what I learned from each activity and (2) how I can apply it to my personal and professional life. The teacher may opt to complete the list if any activities have been overlooked. (It is interesting to note which post-clinical conferences the students did not find memorable!) Reviewing the semester's activities provides a sense of accomplishment and affords group members an opportunity to evaluate how they might apply the content they learned and the communication skills they developed to their daily lives.

A third termination exercise involves having the group sit in a small circle to share some final positive messages with each other. Each member is asked to tell every other member what she learned from her, or why she enjoyed being in the group with her, or how she feels that person's behavior was helpful to the group. This exercise may be done verbally or anonymously in writing. Our groups usually choose to share verbally. This exercise provides the group members with an opportunity to say, "I like you, and I'll miss you because . . . and goodbye." The students seem to enjoy having the chance to say something personal to each other. Sometimes, there is much laughter during this exercise and occasionally even some tears, but usually the students walk away with a good feeling about themselves and about their fellow group members.

COPING WITH GROUP PROBLEMS

It is not uncommon for a group to have a problem that serves an an obstacle to productive functioning. Even a well-developed group will occasionally run up against an internal problem; therefore, it is helpful if the teacher is aware of the existence of group problems and how they might be dealt with.

Resistance

When a teacher uses group process, she can expect to meet resistance. Resistance may be defined as opposing or fighting against something. Frequently, the source of resistance is change, as change causes stress and threatens a loss of security. Group process is experienced as change; it represents the unknown and often leads to resistance.

Resistance within a group may be mild and barely evident—perhaps only one person manifests resistance; or it may be overwhelming and strong, obvious in the behavior of many or all members. Either way, it needs to be evaluated. Is it transient? Will it subside as security within the person or within the group increases? Is it the first behavioral indication of the existence of a more complex problem? Through experience, the teacher learns to recognize various levels and variations of resistance and to deal with them.

Group resistance may take many forms. The group may resist by being non-productive, disinterested or apathetic. A more aggressive form is intragroup fighting or anger directed toward the teacher. We frequently see subtle resistance demonstrated by an inability or unwillingness by members to "settle down" and begin work on their task assignment. Or the group may begin the assignment and then "run out of gas" before completing it. Occasionally, group members will verbalize their resistance, such as, "We really don't think this assignment is worthwhile."

Similarly; individual resistance may take many forms. The student may simply withdraw and refuse to contribute to the group, or she may become angry about an assignment. Resistance is quite common in early group process sessions, as the students are trying to adjust to a new method of learning. A student might comment "I don't want to talk to other students. I want to learn from the teacher, not from my classmates." This type of early resistance is common and usually transient, disappearing as group process becomes familiar and therefore more acceptable.

Resistance also occurs when an assignment is poorly understood, overwhelmingly unrealistic or threatening. On one occasion, when a group was assigned the task of keeping a diary or log of their reactions and feelings as they read a particular book, resistance among all members ran high. The students were aware that this assignment was only being done by their group as a trial. They were willing to participate in this trial, but not to the extent of such a long assignment. The teacher acknowledged the resistance and asked the group to discuss it and come up with a way of handling the situation that seemed fair and acceptable to them. Participation was high in the discussion that followed. About twenty minutes was allowed for this discussion. Ultimately, the students changed the mandatory two pages of log per chapter of text to an optional number of pages, and moved the due date until after vacation instead of before it. The teacher was surprised and pleased with their decision, having anticipated that they might refuse the assignment totally! Following their discussion, resistance to this assignment became nonexistent. Each completed the assignment fully and on time.

On another occasion, the teacher asked students to present and discuss in a triad situation an actual personal or professional problem or concern. In one triad, a student talked about her difficulty in sharing herself in a group situation and how uncomfortable she felt. Another shared a breakdown in communication that had occurred that morning with her husband and her feelings of disappointment and anger. The third manifested signs of resistance. In a joking manner, she presented the problem of her cap falling off while giving nursing care. At the close of the exercise, she said to the teacher, "This whole thing was silly. I can't manufacture problems." This student was unable to share a personal part of herself with the group, found the assignment threatening and resisted genuine participation by offering a non-threatening superficial problem.

As resistance is common, the teacher needs to recognize its various forms and assess its significance. In dealing with it, she needs to encourage the student or students to recognize, verbalize and examine their resistive feelings and behavior. At times she may need to help a whole group recognize this behavior and identify the motivation behind it. Her intervention often takes the same form as it does for other group problems, and should be carried out using appropriate feedback and communication skills. Most often, the intervention can be accomplished within the group. On occasion, however, it is beneficial to deal with an individual's resistance in a private teacher-student conference. At other times, such as in the beginning developmental stages of group process, resistance may subside on its own without intervention. It is the teacher who must discriminate between the forms of resistance, its meaning to the group and the most appropriate form of intervention.

Intervention within the Group. If the teacher determines that intervention is necessary for resistance or any other problem, as discussed earlier in the problem confrontation stage of group development, she must first make the group members aware of the existence of the problem, and then help them determine what is causing it. This is important, because the teacher as observer may be aware of a problem long before the group members are. She may observe behavioral changes such as resistance to task assignment or to the teacher, group anger or increased intragroup conflict. She may decide it is necessary to stop group activity and offer some feedback. This feedback usually is given as a statement of observation and a question of cause, for example, "I've noticed your group is having difficulty getting started with the task assignment. I wonder what is causing this." Once the teacher has pointed out the existence of a problem and described its behavioral components, the group members should be encouraged to discuss and further define the problem and explore its causes. They will respond more favorably to the task of solving their problem if they are allowed to analyze its causes and come up with solutions by themselves, rather than having the teacher tell them what to do.

In addition to direct teacher feedback, we also use the mechanism of self-feedback through our group evaluation form. Regardless of the way it is offered, feedback is necessary to point out the existence of a problem and to initiate constructive group discussion regarding it.

Monopolizing

The purpose of group process is for the group members to share their ideas, learn from each other and contribute to all group decisions and outcomes. If one or two members control the majority of conversation, the group process purpose is not served.

It is common for a group to have one or two persons who talk excessively. If one person is doing all the talking, only one viewpoint is being expressed, and other members are cheated of the opportunity to share their thoughts and feelings. This frequently leads to irritation, anger or hostility. If the situation persists, often the anger reaches the point where it is destructively expressed on a verbal or behavioral level, or the group members settle into an apathetic state allowing the monopolizer to prattle on and assume responsibility for the group.

We have observed examples of situations in which the group members themselves acknowledged the problem and handled it successfully. In one instance, in a five-member group there were two monopolizers who competed constantly for "center stage." Eventually, these two students were talking just to each other while the three others sat silently and listened. Finally, one afternoon the three silent members joined forces and came to conference prepared to deal with the monopolizers. On receiving the assignment, one of the silent members spoke up, "I really have done a lot of research for today's conference, and I would like to share what I've learned. I'd also like to know what everyone else learned. Maybe we could take turns talking so everyone gets a chance; also, if one person talks at a time, we could all listen to what they're saying." This was a positive, tactful way to handle the problem without causing anyone to "lose face."

In another situation there was a single monopolizer who totally dominated all discussions. She felt the need to have all members concur with her opinions and kept restating them to drive them home. Whenever another member stated a differing thought, the monopolizer would quickly interrupt with, "No, you don't understand what I mean. Let me explain it again." The other group members found it very difficult to silence her. They did not want to offend her because they liked her, but they became progressively more irritated and resented being told they "didn't understand." The instructor gave the group the group evaluation form with hopes of bringing the problem to light. As they settled down to discuss their answers to the questionnaire, the monopolizer, as usual, took over:

Carol: Well, question number one is "Did you have a chance to talk as much as you wanted to?" I guess we all put 'yes" for that one.
Judy: No! I put "no."
Beth: So did I.
Carol: What? [laughing] You're kidding. I always get to say all I want to.
Judy: Yes, *you* do. [moment of silence]
Carol: You mean you don't get to talk because I talk too much?
Sandy: Well, I appreciate your ideas, Carol, but usually I have some thoughts I'd like to express too, and they might be interesting to you also.
Carol: Gee, I just thought you all didn't want to talk so I figured I had to carry the ball.
Judy: I think we'd all get more out of it if we carried the ball together.
Carol (laughing): Right, I get the point, I'm glad you told me, I really didn't

realize I was talking too much. Next time I do, give me some sort of a signal.

Beth: Okay. I'll put my hand over your mouth. [much laughter from whole group]

In this situation, the teacher provided the tool to expose the problem, and the group handled it well. This was a close, productive group that had run into a temporary problem, but the members were secure enough as a group to confront it honestly and openly.

Sometimes, the group is unable to deal with the monopolizer and with their own feelings toward her. In this instance, direct teacher intervention may be necessary. The teacher might intervene by simply saying, "That's very interesting, Carol. I wonder how the rest of you feel about what Carol said." This might quiet down the overtalkative student.

If the student is unaware that she is a monopolizer, a more direct approach on the teacher's part may be necessary. 'I've noticed that Carol does most of the talking in this group, and it appears that the rest of you allow her to assume total responsibility." This type of approach lays the responsibility for dealing with the problem on the total group rather than any one person.

It is important to remember that the monopolizer often does not realize she is dominating the conversation. She may not be aware of her behavior and how it is affecting the group members. The teacher's intervention goal must be to help each student recognize the effects of monopolistic behavior on the group and develop ways to modify it.

Silence

The silent group is most frustrating to the teacher. It is important to determine the reason for the silence. Sometimes, silence within the group is desirable, such as following a significant interchange or a discussion of death or separation. Silence in the orientation stage is common, as the group members are often anxious and insecure about the group and themselves.

Sometimes, silence indicates the group members' feelings toward the task assignment. They may find it overwhelming and threatening, or irrelevant; or they may simply need more direction before they can begin. In this instance, it may be necessary for the teacher and group members to discuss the objectives and goals of the assignment, and determine whether they can in fact be met. We have found that silence in a formerly productive group often reflects this situation.

Group silence might also occur following an angry interchange and be indicative of hidden anger. It is best not to allow this type of silence to continue very long. It may be necessary for the teacher to intervene and encourage group problem confrontation. She might do this by saying, "You seem to be very quiet over here. Would someone care to comment on the silence?" For the most part, it is usually better for the teacher to make this observation and not intervene further. Ultimately, someone will speak, usually the person who is most uncomfortable with silence.

Perhaps more significant than group silence is the silence of an individual group member. "Individual silence may mean that the person is holding back information or self in order to punish the group or the leader, that he may fear displeasing others, that he is in agreement, or that he is trying to escape talking because he is anxious." [10, p. 45] .

All of the meanings of silence for the group may also be applied to the individual member as well. Sometimes, individual silence is caused by negative past group experience, as when a member spoke out and was ridiculed or attacked by other group members. We have found that using diads and triads early and frequently often helps silent members feel more secure about speaking out.

Apathy

Group apathy is also an unnerving experience for the teacher. The apathetic group appears bored and disinterested. Discussions seem to be disjointed and purposeless. Members arrive late, leave early and rush through their task assignment with the major part of their energies spent on clock-watching.

Group apathy frequently, but not always, stems from one of two causes: (1) the teacher's style of leadership or (2) the group's negative viewpoint of the assigned task. Occasional apathy is probably nothing to be concerned about. We see it often near the end of a semester or just before a vacation period. However, continued group apathy requires direct intervention to determine the cause. If the teacher suspects her leadership may be the problem, she should check out the student's responses to her, e.g., "I've noticed the group seems quiet and uninvolved. I wonder if you are responding to the way I'm doing things?" or "I wonder if you have some feelings about the task assignment that you would like to share?" Another approach might be, 'I've noticed the group doesn't seem very interested in the assignment. Can anyone suggest a different way for us to accomplish our learning objective for today?" This approach encourages direct student involvement, which fosters commitment that will alleviate apathy.

In dealing with silence and apathy, it is important for the teacher to assist the group to analyze the cause and how to cope with it. Teacher interventions should not only deal with the current problem, but serve as guidelines to the group as to how they might handle it on their own should it occur again.

Emotional Outbursts

It is rare for group members to lose control during a task-oriented group process session. The group does not exist to display feelings, but rather offers opportunity to explore them, the motivations behind them and their possible effect on behavior. Group norms usually disapprove of uncontrolled emotional outbursts, but this does not mean that they will not occur occasionally. Often, group discussions touch on issues of great significance to the students and feelings may run high. An emotional outburst may occur especially from a student who perhaps has less control than others. One student s uncontrolled outburst is often indicative of a high level of feeling running through the group.

We have found that the most common emotional outbursts in our groups involve feelings of anger, sadness or being emotionally overwhelmed. Anger may occur between two members who have strong opposing feelings on an issue. Occasionally, an outburst may occur on a larger scale when a group has difficulty handling conflict. If anger is not acknowledged and handled constructively, tension builds, more anger is generated and the group breaks down into opposing subgroups. In this instance, hostility runs high and precludes productivity. Frequently, an outburst of crying may occur when a group member is personally touched by a situation or is emotionally overwhelmed. Generally, group reaction to an emotional outburst is embarrassment, silence and withdrawal. Two components emerge here: the individual who lost control needs to be supported as she is usually embarrassed and acutely aware of the group's negative response to her outburst; and the group members need to examine their responsive feeling and behavior and learn positive and constructive ways of exploring the here and now meaning behind the outburst. Since an emotional outburst is indicative of high feeling within the entire group rather than just the feelings of one member, it is essential not only to explore its basis promptly and thoroughly but also to identify similar feelings in other group members.

The teacher's first intervention needs to be concerned with the individual or individuals directly involved. Reflective feedback often clarifies the emotion and provides an opportunity for discussing it. The teacher might say, "You sound very angry, Lynn; let's talk about it." This type of intervention is supportive in that it recognizes and accepts the individual's emotional state and expresses a desire to help. A similar statement may be made to a crying person, perhaps accompanied by a physical gesture such as a comforting touch.

After acknowledging the outburst, the teacher can help clarify its meaning. It is often helpful to recall the events that precipitated the response, for example, "You seemed to become upset while discussing Sally and Cynthia's response to your patient's behavior." The teacher might further offer a possible analysis based on her observations of the group's interaction. "I wonder if you sense the group is being judgmental toward your patient." The teacher needs to be supportive and encourage the student to explore her feelings to help clarify the meaning of the outburst. The teacher's accepting, concerned attitude serves as a role model for the group members. They are guided toward examining the situation rather than withdrawing from it.

When the teacher has been supportive and has encouraged the individual to clarify her feelings, she can then involve the group in the experience. She might say, "Lynn has been sharing her reactions with us. I wonder if some of you would like to share your feelings with Lynn and the group." This type of intervention helps pull the group back together again and reduce its separation from the member who has had the outburst. The outburst then becomes a shared experience, and the group is encouraged to approach it as a group problem that requires collective understanding and input in order to be resolved. Successful intervention helps the group learn how to deal effectively with these situations. In the long run, open examination of the meaning and precipitating factors behind an outburst decreases their occurrence.

Whether dealing with group problems or assisting a group through its developmental stages, the teacher must possess and use four critical factors: genuine care and concern for the group members and their functioning together; knowledge of group process concepts and theories; development of communication skills necessary for constructive intervention; and awareness of one's impact on the group process[23].

In Chapter 6, we will present some actual confluent activities that we have employed in our endeavors to facilitate cognitive and affective learning through group process.

REFERENCES

1. Aspy, D. *Toward a Technology for Humanizing Education.* Champaign, Illinois: Research Press, 1972.
2. Aspy, D. Toward a Technology Which Helps Teachers Humanize Their Classrooms. *Educational Leadership* Research Supplement 29:626–628, 1971.
3. Bates, M., and Johnson, C. *Group Leadership.* Denver, Colo.: Love, 1972.
4. Benne, K. D., and Sheats, P. Functional Roles of Group Members. *Journal of Social Issues* 4(2):41–49, 1948.
5. Bogad, S. Process in the Classroom. In G. I. Brown; T. Yeomans; and L. Grizzard (Eds.), *The Live Classroom.* New York: Viking, 1975.
6. Capuzzi, D. Information Intermix: An Approach to Group Guidance. *Journal of Reading* 16:453–458, 1973.
7. Carkhuff, R. *Helping and Human Relations.* New York: Holt, 1969.
8. Carkhuff, R., and Berenson, B. *Beyond Counseling and Therapy.* New York: Holt, 1967.
9. Clark, C. *The Nurse as Group Leader.* New York: Springer, 1977.
10. Clark, C. Simulation gaming: A new teaching strategy in nursing education. *Nurse Educator* 1(4): 4–9, 1976.
11. Egan, G. *The Skilled Helper.* Monterey, Calif.: Brooks/Cole, 1975.
12. Egan, G. *You and Me: The Skills of Communicating and Relating to Others.* Monterey, Calif.: Brooks Cole, 1977.
13. Evans, R. *Carl Rogers, The Man and His Ideas.* New York: Dutton, 1975.
14. Gazda, G.; Asbury, F.; Balzer, F.; Childers, W.; and Walters, R. *Human Relations Development: Manual for Educators* (2nd ed.). Boston: Allyn and Bacon, 1977.
15. Guralnik, D. (Ed.). *Webster's New World Dictionary of the American Language.* New York: William Collins and World, 1972.
16. James, M., and Jongeward, D. *Born to Win: Transactional Analysis with Gestalt Experiments.* Reading, Mass.: Addison-Wesley, 1971.
17. Kauffman, M. On developing empathy: Sharing the patient's experience. *American Journal of Nursing* 78:860–861, 1978.
18. King, V. A confluent approach to nursing education through group process. *Nurse Educator* 3(3):20–25, 1978.
19. Lefrancois, G. *Psychology for Teaching* (2nd ed.). Belmont, Calif.: Wadsworth, 1975.
20. Lincoln, R.; Layton, J.; and Holdman, H. Using simulated patients to teach assessment. *Nursing Outlook* 26:316–320, 1978.
21. Patterson, C. *Humanistic Education.* Englewood Cliffs, N.J.: Prentice-Hall, 1973.
22. Rogers, C. *Freedom to Learn.* Columbus, Ohio: Charles E. Merrill, 1969.
23. Sampson, E., and Marthas, M. *Group Process for the Health Professions.* New York: Wiley, 1977.
24. Schmuck, R., and Schmuck, P. *Group Process in the Classroom.* Dubuque, Iowa: Wm. C. Brown Company, 1971.
25. Shostrom, E. *Man, the Manipulator.* Nashville, Tenn.: Abingdon, 1967.
26. Stanford, G. *Developing Effective Classroom Groups.* New York: Hart, 1977.
27. Stanford, G., and Roark, A. *Human Interaction in Education.* Boston: Allyn and Bacon, 1974. Available from Dr. Gene Stanford, Children's Hospital, 219 Bryant Street, Buffalo, N.Y. 14222.
28. Wackman, D.; Miller, S.; and Nunnally, E. *Alive and Aware.* Minneapolis: Interpersonal Communication Programs, 1976.

CHAPTER 6

The "How To" of Group Process

The examples of our confluent approach in this chapter reflect our interest in facilitating the total growth of students toward self-actualization and re-sponsibility. Through the learning activities described here, students become increasingly aware of their behavior, not why they are behaving in a particular way, but rather what they are doing and how they are experiencing it. Their mastery of cognitive content is an integral part of that growth.

Each of these examples involves experiential learning activities. The quality of personal involvement is special. Rogers[3] describes how the whole per-son—intellectual and emotional—is part of an experiential learning event. Al-though the stimulus may come from the outside, (i.e., through group task assignments), the experience for the individual student is self-initiated. The sense of discovery, searching and understanding comes from within. "It makes a difference in the behavior, the attitudes, perhaps even the personality of the learner"[3, p. 5]. Through these experiential activities, we have observed stu-dents evaluate their experience, know whether it has helped them to learn what they want to know and set spontaneously their own new goals for learning.

These examples are "person-centered" rather than being didactic and con-centrating on the teaching of skills, disciplines or subject matter. They are learning activities in which there is a flowing together of mind and feelings. During these activities, there is dynamic interplay between the students. They become involved and committed to each other and their group. According to Stanford and Roark[4], although a student may learn by doing something alone, the meaning of what she learns is realized only through her interaction with others. Accordingly, these learning activities within the setting of group process foster dynamic interaction. They have enabled us to implement human-istic nursing education on a continuing basis.

Each semester we develop new activities and observe how well they accomplish the goal of confluence. There is some variation in how well the activities work, with differences occurring from group to group and from year to year. Often, their effectiveness depends on the stage of the group's development.

To demonstrate the diversity available with this approach, we have selected a sample of activities that we have found to be reasonably effective. When available, we have included student dialogue obtained from tapes of the learning sessions and instructor logs.

EXERCISE 1 : PHARMACOLOGY PRE-CLINICAL CONFERENCE – ANTIARRHYTHMIC DRUGS

Objectives–Cognitive

Students will
1. Discuss the route of electrical current through the heart.
2. Define the following terms: sinus rhythm, nodal rhythm and automaticity.
3. Define the following pharmacological drug actions: inotropic (positive and negative), chronotropic, dromotropic and pressor.
4. Describe the action of cardiac depressants (procainamide, quinidine, lidocaine) on the heart and the specific arrhythmias each one is used to treat.
5. Discuss the side effects that procainamide, quinidine and lidocaine have in common on the heart.
6. Explain the rationale behind nursing responsibilities listed in the textbook in relation to antiarrhythmic therapy.
7. List and discuss the two mechanisms by which propranolol exerts an antiarrhythmic effect on the heart.
8. Explain the use of digitalis as an antiarrhythmic agent.

Objectives–Affective

Student will
1. Share feelings related to assignment.
2. Be responsible for own individual and other group members' learning.

Confluent Techniques

Support groups of five students.

Pre-clinical Conference, 30 minutes

1. (1–2 minutes) Allow students this time to glance over their notes from the previously assigned chapter reading. Then ask them to put away their notes. Conversation is more spontaneous when they do not read from their notes or the book.

2. (15–18 minutes) Assign groups the task of discussing the cognitive objectives listed. Write these objectives on the blackboard before class or pass out one typed copy to each group.
3. (10 minutes) Give one copy of the pharmacology quiz to each group. Each group of five students participates as a unit in taking the quiz.

Usually students complete the quiz in about five minutes. Depending on the time available, answers are compared between the two groups, or each individual group may correct its own quiz, with members seeking whatever assistance may be necessary from each other and the instructor to ensure understanding of correct answers.

Handouts: Sample Quiz

ANTIARRYTHMIA DRUG QUIZ*

True/False
1. All cardiac arrhythmias require drug therapy.
2. Some arrhythmias can be controlled with the use of mild tranquilizers.
3. An ectopic beat is that originating anywhere but in the S.A. node.
4. Propranolol tends to produce other than cardiac side effects.
Calculation
Dilantin, 250 mg I.V. push is ordered. The medication vial is labeled 50 mg in 2 cc. How many cc will you give?
Multiple Choice
1. Which of the following may be a symptom of quinidine toxicity?
   a. urticaria
   b. tremor
   c. muscular pain
   d. tinnitus
   e. blindness
2. Lidocaine is used intravenously to:
   a. increase peripheral circulation
   b. decrease damage to the myocardium
   c. slow the heart
   d. decrease ventricular irritability during diastole

---

*Adapted from: Ralston, S., and Hale, M. *Review and Application of Clinical Pharmacology.* Philadelphia: Lippincott, 1977.

3. The drug used most often to treat atrial fibrillation is:
   a. digitalis
   b. quinidine
   c. sodium nitrate
   d. papaverine
   e. epinephrine
4. The drug that is the best choice for treatment in prevention of ventricular fibrillation is:
   a. quinidine
   b. procaine
   c. digitalis
   d. lidocaine
   e. isoproterenol
5. If a patient receiving an anticoagulant is started on diphenylhydantoin sodium for arrhythmias, what adjustment should be made in the dosage of the anticoagulant?
   a. it should be reduced
   b. it should be increased
   c. it should be discontinued
   d. no change is necessary
6. Which of the following antiarrhythmic drugs is a beta blocking agent?
   a. quinidine
   b. procainamide hydrochloride
   c. lidocaine hydrochloride
   d. propranolol hydrochloride

Comments

The pharmacology pre-clinical conferences have received extremely positive evaluations from students. They like having weekly time allotted for structured discussion of pertinent and specific pharmacology. They are responsible for making the discussion worthwhile, and they handle it well.

As students are sharing information, you will hear them also talking about their misunderstandings of the information, their confusion, and their feelings of being frustrated and overwhelmed by the complexity and the amount of information to learn. They seem to see the quizzes as tools by which they can evaluate their areas of strength and weakness.

Often members of the group will ask to photocopy the objectives and the quiz. They take turns doing this and share copies with the rest of their group, using them to prepare and study for course examinations.

All of the following examples in the chapter are of exercises used in post-clinical conference.

EXERCISE 2: GENERAL ORIENTATION TO GROUP PROCESS

Objectives—Cognitive

Students will
1. Develop a beginning knowledge of group process, the teacher's role and the student's role.
2. Review SOLER listening skills[1].

Objectives—Affective

Students will
1. Share feelings about beginning of the semester.
2. Select and talk about meaningful learning experiences of the day.
3. Begin development of trust as a foundation for relationship with peers.

Objectives—Psychomotor

Students will practice SOLER listening skills[1].

Confluent Techniques

Diad; support group of five students; discussion group of ten students.

Description

1. (3 minutes) Introduce group process concept to group of ten students. "We are going to be using a different format in our pre-clinical and post-clinical conferences this semester. It is a group process approach. I will not be leading, directing or controlling the conferences. Instead, you will be responsible for sharing your individual preparation, learning and experiences with each other in pairs, small groups of three to five students, and sometimes in our larger group of ten students. You will be doing most of the talking, discussing and sharing. This approach is based on the philosophy that the most important person to an individual's learning is the individual; second in importance is the individual's peers or classmates; third is the library; fourth, maybe, is the teacher.
    "You may be wondering what I will be doing if I am not directly going to lead

and control the conference discussions. I will be responsible for planning the discussion assignments and activities for the groups. I will also, not at first, but soon, alternate between groups, taking a limited part in your discussions as a group member. In addition, I will be a resource person for areas related to medical-surgical nursing, communication skills and group development. I will be pleased now to answer any questions and listen to concerns that you have about the way the clinical conferences will be handled."

2. (5–10 minutes) Allow time for initial student responses and questions. Responses are usually mixed. Illustration:

—"This sounds okay. I don't mind working in groups."
—"I don't think I'm going to like this. You are the most important person here. You are the expert. You should lead the discussions."
—"Why don't we select one person to present a patient's case to the entire group each week. That way we would all benefit."
—I'll try it."

3. (5 minutes) Divide the group of ten students into two groups of five. Position the groups as far apart as possible. Otherwise, the discussion noise will interfere with the ability of students to hear each other.

4. (10 minutes) Ask students to discuss and make a group list of good listening behaviors. At the end of seven or eight minutes, have students share, discuss and contrast the lists from the two groups within the larger one.

5. (5 minutes) Review SOLER[1] with the students. Write it on the blackboard for reference.

S–face the person squarely
O–keep an open posture
L–lean toward the other person
E–maintain eye contact
R–be relaxed

6. (5 minutes) Direct students to find a partner for a diad activity. When they have paired off, continue to give directions. Ask them to discuss with their partner something they learned during their first week of clinical experience that is important to them, and to practice SOLER attending skills during this activity.

7. (5 minutes) Have students repeat the above activity with a new partner. They may discuss the same experience they discussed with their first partner, or select a different one.

8. (1-2 minutes) Request students to form one large circle.

9. (15 minutes) Assign discussion task: "You have had a little experience now with how we will be working together this semester. Would you please

share your reactions to this experience with each other." Instructor may remain as part of the circle participating when she decides it is appropriate to do so. It is the responsibility of the instructor to terminate the class on time.

Sample Dialogue

G: I liked the group discussion, but I felt uncomfortable in the one-to-one.

B: I didn t like the one-to-one. It's okay if I talk with my patients. That's important and worthwhile. But I didn't learn anything when I was talking to a classmate.

S: It's good though to be aware of what you are doing. You could be turning someone off and not know it. I'm learning to be more aware of what I'm doing. That's helpful.

W: Well, that's what this is about. Isn't it? Learning with each other; practicing skills that will help us with our patients.

B: I'm not learning this way. I'm not interested in listening to my classmates. I'm not learning anything. It can be quite boring.

G: I'm not sure I want to look forward to 14 weeks of 20 minutes of one-to-one talking. I'd be afraid of that. I wouldn't like that.

B: I'm not sure if I've made myself clear.

D: I liked listening. I liked trying to concentrate on what was being said.

B: Not me! I won't mention names, but earlier today I deliberately let a class-mate who was boring me know that I didn't want to listen. I did not want to hear her, and I'm sure I let her know that.

Instructor (to B): I'm hearing that listening to patients is of more value to you right now.

B: Yes.

M (to B): I wonder if it is because you are going to do something with the information, give pain medication or get something for them or report their problem.

T (to M): Yes, you have to listen to patients, make an assessment or a judg-ment, considering what they are saying. That's really important.

B: I suppose that's part of it. I do care more about patients. It's important and interesting to listen to them.

Instructor (to B): I'd like to go back to something that you said earlier about knowing you were not listening to a classmate and giving her signs that you didn't want to hear. You indicated that you were aware of your behavior and aware of what you were feeling. That is good. Awareness of each of these is important, but I'd like to talk for a minute specifically about awareness of feelings. It's essential to know and process what you are feeling as you are listening to someone and to be aware of how this is influencing your behavior. Awareness and acceptance of your feelings at any given moment is called being congruent. This is also connected to what one of you said about learning to be more aware of your own behavior and how it is affecting others. The more aware we are of our feelings, the more congruent we can be. New awareness about ourselves, about our feelings about our behavior, is something we might gain through this kind of practice and sharing. It can be risky, though, even if we like what we learn.

B: And we might want to change our behavior.

Instructor: Yes, and that is up to you, if you choose to do that. But for now, let's close considering that we might learn something we like!

Comments

Resistance in this beginning session is demonstrated in the dialogue of B and G, and in the silence of three members who chose not to participate verbally. B is rather angry and frightened, hence even more resistive than G. It is evident that most members need to improve their communication skills. For example, B, who was the most vocal, revealed a need to become more aware of the effects of her behavior on others and aware of her immediate feelings.

During this beginning conference, the instructor attempted to set an open, fairly positive, nonjudgmental tone for the group conference that would alleviate some anxiety and provide an opportunity for sharing of attitudes and feelings. Attitudes and opinions were shared. It was not until later conferences that the students felt comfortable enough openly to identify and share feelings.

EXERCISE 3: SOAP NOTING

Objectives—Cognitive

Students will

1. Contrast normal and abnormal levels of pediatric infant growth and development.
2. Apply principles of nursing process in developing immediate and long-range nursing intervention with specific behavioral objectives for pediatric patient with developmental deficiencies.
3. Demonstrate principles of POMR in recording data for specific patient problems.
4. Compare and critique SOAP notes for specified patient problems.
5. Describe feelings that might be observed in parents of afflicted child.
6. Review specifics of anemia, upper respiratory infection and Down's syndrome, i.e. cause, medical treatment and nursing intervention for patient and family.

Objectives—Affective

Students will

1. Share feelings about learning experience.
2. Reach consensus about nursing care plan and SOAP notes.

Objective—Psychomotor

Students will

1. Write SOAP notes for specified patient problems.
2. Write immediate and long-term nursing care plan for specified patient problems.

Confluent Techniques

Support groups of five students; intergroup discussion.

Class Preparation

Assign SOAP Noting handout to students a few days before the exercise is to be
used in conference. Ask the students to follow the directions in the exercise and
bring the completed form with them to conference to use in a discussion with
their group members. Assign additional POMR reading for review. Suggest
students use any other review that seems appropriate for helping them to deal
with the nursing aspects of the patient's medical-surgical problems.

Post-clinical Conference: SOAP Noting

1. (1–2 minutes) Divide group of ten students into their usual support groups.
2. (30 minutes) Assign students the task of reaching a consensus in each group
   for appropriate answers to POMR exercise—cue lists, problem lists, SOAP
   notes with nursing care plan. As instructor, move freely back and forth between the groups, participating as a member in relation to the exercise and
   intervening as observer, resource person and model, as needed.
3. (10–15 minutes) Direct the two groups to share their work and reach an agreement on one combined, appropriate response to the exercise.
4. (5–10 minutes) Ask students to share with each other some of the feelings
   they had during this learning experience.

Handouts for SOAP Noting Exercise.*

Directions: SOAP Noting (student's copy)
Please read the following case history and complete the exercises as directed using the principles of POMR with which you are familiar.

Medical History
An eight-month-old girl with Down's syndrome is admitted for treatment of an upper respiratory infection. The baby became ill six days ago with a "runny nose and cough." Coryza nonpurulent. Temperature ranges from 99° to 102° F. Ampicillin started two days ago; aspirin (gr 1½) used to control fever; no improvement noted. Parents having difficulty getting child to swallow oral ampicillin. Baby has been breast-fed since birth; refuses spoon, bottle nipples and all solid foods. Heart murmur noted and reported to mother when baby was one month of age; no overt symptoms of cardiac problems.

Physical examination
T 100.8° F (rectal); P 100 (apical); R 28, not labored. Harsh, frequent non-productive cough; rales and diminshed breath sounds left chest. Flushed face. Skin color, pale. Resists approach by strangers. Has typical Down's facies, tongue protrusion, some drooling noted. Tests (Denver Developmental Screening Test) at 3- to 4-month level for gross and fine motor development, and at a 2- to 3-month level in language and social skills. Poor head control; likes supine position. In hypotonic "pithed frog" position at rest.

Laboratory data
  white blood cell count 18,500
  hematocrit 30%
  hemoglobin 10.5 Gm%
  urine normal
  electrolytes normal

Instructions
From the history, physical examination record and the laboratory values reported, select all of the cues that will help identify the patient's problems and list them in the space provided.
CUE LIST
Medical history

---

*Adapted from: Woolley, F.; Warnick, M.; Kane, R.; and Dyer, E. *Problem-oriented Nursing.* New York: Springer, 1974, pp. 110–119.

Physical examination

Laboratory data

Now, using your cues, develop a problem list for this patient. Place all cues under a problem.
PROBLEM LIST
DATE   NUMBER   PROBLEM

For exercise in planning nursing intervention and in writing SOAP progress notes, write initial progress notes for each of the patient's temporary or permanent problems that you have identified and that are currently active.

Please bring this activity sheet with you to conference to discuss with your group members.

SOAP Noting (instructor's copy—includes case history)

CUE LIST
Medical history
    runny nose
    cough
    elevated temperature
    Down's syndrome—retarded development indicated by Denver Developmental
      Screening Test (DDST)
    breast-fed, refuses bottle nipples
    refuses solid foods and spoon

Physical examination
    cough—harsh; nonproductive
    flushed face
    pale skin color
    resists strangers

facial characteristics of Down's syndrome
well nourished and well hydrated
T 100.8° F—rectal
R 28—not labored
diminished breath sounds with rales
poor head control
hypotonic "pithed frog" position at rest
Laboratory data
    white blood cell count 18,500
    hematocrit 30%
    hemoglobin 10.5 Gm%
PROBLEM LIST

DATE	NUMBER	PROBLEM
10/25/73	1	*Down's Syndrome*
		Retarded development indicated by DDST
		Facial characteristics
		Hypotonic "pithed frog" position at rest
		Refuses solid food and spoon
		Refuses bottle-feeding
		Poor head control
10/25/73	2	*Anemia*
		Hematocrit 30%
		Hemoglobin 10.5 Gm%
		Refuses solid food
		Breast-feeding only
		Pale skin color
10/25/73	3	*Upper respiratory infection*
		Cough
		Flushed face
		Temperature 100.5° F—rectal
		Respiration 28, not labored
		Decreased breath sounds with rales
		Runny nose
		White blood cell count 18,500

SOAP NOTES:
Temporary Problem: Upper Respiratory Infection
S Mother states child has had "runny nose" and cough for six days
    Temperature between 99° and 102° F
    Ampicillin started two days ago

O Child coughing now; cough harsh and frequent
   Nonpurulent drainage from nose; face flushed
   T 100.8°F; WBC 18,500
A URI not improving
P 1. Croupette with cold mist and O_2. Use large infant seat (e.g., Starr-
       Rider) in croupette.
   2. Use dropper for ampicillin.
   3. If not able to give ampicillin orally, notify physician.
   4. Mother to breast-feed child on demand. Place cot in room.

Permanent Problem: Down's syndrome

S Child refuses spoon, solid foods, and bottle nipples; has been breast-fed
   since birth.
O Retardation indicated by DDST (2- to 3-month level language and social
   skills and 3- to 4-month level gross and fine motor development).
A Management of Down's syndrome inadequate.
P Establish formal times to spend with parents and teach them skills to help
   manage child's problems. Teach parents:
   1. Keep child on stomach as much as possible. Work into this gradually,
       placing her on stomach several times daily (8-12-4-8). Gradually in-
       crease time and number of placements. Use a small hand mirror propped
       up in front of her to keep her attention; encourage her to lift up her
       head and reach out in front to play. Use small, bright, noisy toys to
       hold her attention while in this position.
   2. Begin immediately with "pretend" spoon feedings. Place a small spoon
       firmly on the center of her tongue and press down slightly. Use empty
       spoon 3 to 4 days. Then begin with a medium-thick rice cereal and
       milk preparation. Encourage to swallow before giving more. If neces-
       sary, gently close lower jaw to reinforce the idea of shutting mouth to
       produce swallowing. Always feed from the midline, with child directly
       in front.
   3. Pull child to sitting position several times following each diaper change.

Anemia

O Hct 30; Hgb 10.5; T 100.8°F; skin color pale
   Breast-fed; no supplemental foods
A Anemia; aggravated by inability to maintain dietary balance; further com-
   plicated by current URI
P 1. Use plan indicated for Down's syndrome and URI.
   2. Consult physician on $FeSO_4$ supplement.
   3. Check Hct in one month.

Comments

This exercise has been offered during a post-clinical conference at the beginning of the fall semester of the students' second year. It provides a structured and fairly thorough review of POMR, which most of the students seem to need at this point. In addition, the content of this case study fits our curriculum needs, which at this time concern the hospitalized child and problems related to oxygen deprivation. The content of the case study can be adjusted to fit the particular cognitive structure of any curriculum.

An instructor's guide to this exercise is offered, as it is especially helpful to ensure that all students are achieving a reasonably similar standard of outcome. It has been interesting to note that most of the student groups add sections to the nursing intervention on meeting the affective needs of the parents. They assume these needs are present, although not included in the data provided.

This learning activity offers a stimulating and enjoyable introduction to dealing with group process in post-clinical conference.

EXERCISE 4: DIABETES DIET THERAPY POST-CLINICAL CONFERENCE

Objectives—Cognitive

Students will
1. Calculate an individualized diet based own dietary needs and principles of diet therapy as a means of controlling diabetes.
2. Discuss aspects of individualized diet in relation to insulin, exercise and weight control.

Objectives—Affective

Students will
1. Compare reactions of various patients with diabetes to diet therapy.
2. Discuss own reactions to individualized diabetic diet therapy.

Confluent Techniques

Diad; support groups of five students.

Class Preparation

Assign activities related to diabetic diet therapy to students a week before they are to be used in class. Ask students to follow directions in the exercise and bring the completed assignment with them to use in diad or small group discussions.

Post-clinical Conference

1. (1-2 minutes) Divide the group of ten students into diads. When they have found their partners (someone who is not from their own support group), ask them to decide who is A and who is B.
2. (10 minutes) Ask B to share in five minutes the rationale behind her completed individualized diet assignment, i.e., how she calculated it, adjustments she make in her regular diet, her reactions to it. At the end of five minutes, A and B switch roles, and A shares her dietary assignment.
3. (1-2 minutes) Ask students to return to their support groups.
4. (15 minutes) Direct students to share with each other the principles of diabetic diet therapy that they have learned from the assignment, and their feelings about this type of control.
5. (25 minutes) Ask students to discuss with each other the results of their clinical talks with patients who have diabetes (see handouts). As instructor, move freely back and forth between the groups and diads, participating as a member in relation to the exercise, and intervening as observer, resource person, and model, as needed. Usually your role will be minimal.
6. (5 minutes) Direct students to spend last few minutes sharing their reactions to this learning activity.

Handouts for Diabetes Diet Therapy Post-clinical Conference

Diabetic Diet Assignment Guide

Please follow the directions for this activity, which will serve as a guide to help you plan a diabetic diet for yourself, using the principles of diet therapy as one method of controlling diabetes.

Steps:

1. Keep a record of your food intake for a 48-hour period. Include the individual breakdown of the CHO, FAT and PROTEIN of each food. Total the amounts for each 24-hour period.
2. Weigh yourself. Convert your pounds of body weight to kilograms.
3. Decide whether you are overweight, underweight, or the ideal (desired) weight.

4. Adjust your total daily caloric intake accordingly. Keep in mind the following recommendations:
    a. Weight reduction: 20 cal/kilogram of body weight
    b. Maintenance of ideal weight: 25 cal/kilogram of body weight
    c. Maintenance of ideal weight for active person: 30 cal/kilogram of body weight
    d. Underweight for someone doing heavy work or for growing child: 35 cal/kilogram of body weight

Remember that a decrease in 500 calories/day for a week will usually cause a weight reduction of 1 lb/week.

5. Use the following recommended amounts for daily intake in a diabetic diet: CHO 40%, FAT 40%, PROTEIN 20%.
6. Use your accumulated information to calculate a diabetic diet for yourself for 48 hours. Include the individual breakdown of each food into grams of CHO, FAT, and PROTEIN. Total the amounts.
7. Compare this calculated diabetic diet with your usual diet. What are the major differences?
    a. CHO, FAT and PROTEIN amounts
    b. caloric amount
    c. time of food intake
    d. distribution of calories throughout the day
8. Describe your feelings about this diabetic diet.
9. Hand in this paper on your regular diet and diabetic diet to your clinical instructor. Be ready to discuss your findings in post-clinical conference.

Guide for Discussion of Diabetic Diet with Patients

A. During your clinical experience, please find two patients who have diabetes. Discuss with each patient the following:
    1. How long has he/she had diabetes?
    2. What kind of change, if any, has diet made in his/her life? (Consider social, family, and work aspects.)
    3. How has he/she coped with the diet?
    4. What were the feelings he/she had when first learning about the need for regulating food intake?
    5. How does he/she manage calculating his/her diet?
B. Compare the situations of the two patients.
    1. Kind of diabetes—maturity or youth onset
    2. Type of controls used and patient compliance
    3. Patient's knowledge of the disease
    4. Patient's reaction to diet management
    5. Effectiveness of control of diabetic condition

C. Come prepared to discuss in post-clinical conference what you have learned from these conversations with your patients and your comparison of their situations.

Sample Student Reactions to Individualized Diabetic Diets

—"I don't want to be controlled."
—"I would hate to have to be on this diet."
—"I see the changes I would have to make. It wouldn't be easy for me."
—"I learned so much . . . I got involved."

Comments

Combining the sharing of the individualized diabetic diet assignment with a discussion of patient interviews regarding the diets creates lively group discussions. It personalizes the learning experience, and ultimately provides an effective and stimulating way to learn the principles of diet therapy for controlling diabetes. The discussion often involves student feelings concerning mandatory change and adaptation to it.

EXERCISE 5: HANDS-ON INSULIN POST-CLINICAL CONFERENCE

Objectives—Cognitive
Students will
1. Accurately identify types of short-, intermediate-, and long-acting insulin, the differences in their time of onset, peak action, and duration of effect.
2. Compare signs and symptoms of hypoglycemia and hyperglycemia and methods of prevention and treatment.
3. Explain the Somogyi effect on blood sugar levels and urine test results.
4. Discuss principles to teach patients in regard to:
   a. care of syringe and needle
   b. storage of insulin
   c. selection of injection sites
   d. aseptic and accurate method of preparation and administration of insulin
5. Review principles of insulin coverage:
   a. proper collection of urine by voiding or catheter
   b. situations in which coverage is used
   c. type of insulin used for coverage
6. Compare advantages and disadvantages of various methods of urine testing.

Objectives—Affective

Students will contrast reactions of various patients beginning to learn self-administration of insulin.

Objectives—Psychomotor

Students will
1. Accurately draw up into a syringe a single dose of one kind of insulin, and into a second syringe a combination of a short- and intermediate-acting insulin (using solution with food dye coloring for short-acting insulin).
2. Accurately test urine for sugar and acetone using various kinds of testing methods.

Confluent Techniques

Diad or triad; small groups of five students.

Class preparation

Assign the students to read the chapter on insulin in their pharmacology book a few days before the hands-on post-clinical conference.

Post-clinical Conference

1. (5 minutes) Explain to students that during this conference they will be reviewing and implementing concepts of insulin therapy and urine testing. To help guide them through this activity, five stations with specific directions and needed equipment have been established. Each station has a specific task or series of tasks to be accomplished by each student. Students will work in diads or triads, moving at random from one station to another until they have completed all requirements.
2. (1–2 minutes) Direct students to select a partner and proceed to a station where they will read and follow the directions for completing the tasks at that station.
3. (45 minutes) Encourage students to complete each of the requirements at a particular station thoroughly before moving on to another one. Students in one diad can solicit assistance and information from another diad. Books may be used for reference if needed. Students who have more experience and expertise in one area may become teachers for a number of other students needing assistance. Students need about 45 minutes to complete

effectively all of the station tasks. They keep track of their own time, moving as rapidly as possible through the activities. Notify them when one-half of the class time has elapsed so they may adjust their working time accordingly.

4. (10 minutes) Ask students to return to their support groups. Assign them the task of sharing what they learned about themselves from this experience and some of the feelings they had as they worked together on the tasks.

Handouts

The activities for each station are placed on an individual 5 x 8 card. They are located at five convenient areas of the room.

Station A. Every student should complete each activity.
Draw up: 15 units of regular insulin
1. Check the syringe for bubbles. Why are they significant?
2. Discuss the duration of effect and time of peak action of regular insulin.
3. Explain when and for what reasons regular insulin is used.
Draw up: 5 units of NPH insulin
1. Compare the differences between NPH and regular insulin (four differences).
2. List the types of insulin that can be mixed in one syringe.
3. If you were mixing two insulins in one syringe, determine which one you would draw up first, and the reasons for doing this.

Station B. Every student should complete each activity.
Order reads: 8 a.m. 10 U NPH insulin and 5 U regular insulin
Prepare this medication order in one syringe.
1. Which insulin did you draw up first? What were your reasons?
2. What methods did you use to avoid contamination of the clear bottle?
3. What is the rationale for administering two kinds of insulin? What is their combined effect?

Station C. Every student should complete each activity.
Insulin coverage:
1. Discuss proper methods for collecting urine for testing by voiding and catheter.
2. Test the sample of urine for sugar and acetone using each method of testing. Compare the results of the various testing methods.
3. Where would you record the test results? What is the most accurate way to record urine test results for sugar?

4. Order reads: 8 a.m. 10 U NPH and coverage   1+ – 0

2+ – 5 U

3+ – 5 U

4+ – 10 U

Draw up insulin order based on results of urine you have tested.

a. Compare the peak action times of each of the insulins referred to in this order.

b. At what time might you look for signs of insulin reaction in the patient receiving this medication order?

Station D. Every student should complete each activity.

Role playing: patient-nurse situation

Use the available equipment and provide one-to-one teaching to each other.

1. Teach the patient how to give a self-injection using appropriate principles of asepsis, site selection, and method of injection.
2. Observe the patient's return demonstration.
3. Explain what you would teach this patient regarding:
   a. care of the syringe and needle
   b. storage of insulin
   c. choice of injection sites
   d. allergic reactions to insulin

Station E. Every student should complete each activity.

Discussion (no notes or books unless absolutely necessary!)

Your patient received 10 U NPH and 15 U regular insulin at 8 a.m. At 11:30 a.m. he shows signs of insulin reaction (hypoglycemia).

1. List ten symptoms he might manifest.
2. Describe what your immediate nursing care would be.
3. Explain three ways the patient could avoid a recurrence of this.
4. Explain which insulin was responsible for this patient's reaction.
5. Compare the signs and symptoms of hypoglycemia to those of hyper-glycemia.
6. Discuss rationale for the nursing intervention for prevention and treatment of hyperglycemia.

Comments

This activity creates an atmosphere of lively discussion, questions and answers, and enjoyable exchanges as the students learn about insulin therapy and urine testing as a combined means for controlling diabetes.

EXERCISE 6: SHARING PERSONAL FEELINGS ABOUT CANCER AND CARING FOR PATIENTS WITH CANCER

Objectives—Cognitive

Students will
1. Identify positive as well as negative aspects of cancer therapy.
2. Identify effective ways to counsel patients with cancer.

Objectives—Affective

Students will
1. Share own feelings about cancer and cancer therapy.
2. Share awareness of own feelings about death and dying.

Objectives—Psychomotor

Students will use effective listening and responding skills in group discussions.

Confluent Techniques

Small groups of five students.

Description

1. (1–2 minutes) Have students sit in usual support groups.
2. (1–2 minutes) Ask students to sit quietly for a few minutes to consider their feelings about cancer and to select a word to describe these feelings.
3. (15 minutes) Have students share their feeling words with each other.
4. (30 minutes) Ask students to describe an experience they had in caring for a patient with cancer and some reactions they had during this experience.
5. (10 minutes) Request that students share with each other what they have learned about themselves from this experience.

Sample Dialogue

T: You remember Mr. Kane who has metastatic cancer of the bladder?
   Group members: (Nod their heads, yes.)
T: Well, yesterday, when I went to say goodbye to Mr. Kane, Dr. R was having a conference with him and his wife. He was giving Mr. Kane a choice between having chemotherapy or not having it. I didn't go into the room because they were having such a serious talk that I didn't want to interrupt.

M: That's pretty tough news to have to hear.

T: Yes, and the medication may cause him to lose his hair or his hearing and even to have cardiac problems. Well, I was up all night thinking about him. Also, I didn't know what I would say to him. I spent a lot of time thinking about that too! I finally decided not to mention either the therapy or the decision. Yet I wanted to let him talk about it if he wanted to, so I said, "Good morning, Mr. Kane. I came in to say goodbye yesterday, but I didn't want to interrupt you. You were having a discussion with Dr. R and your wife." Mr. Kane said to me, "Oh, that would have been okay. You could have come in. He was just telling me about the treatment plan that I had to decide on. I don't have any choice really. Even with the treatment, I have only a 50-50 chance of surviving. And my hair is all going to fall out. What can I do? I decided to have the medication. It's going to start on Monday, so they're going to let me go home for the weekend. Then, I'll return on Monday for the first treatment."

G: It sounds like what you said worked! He talked a lot, like he was anxious for you to hear what was happening to him. And you didn't ask any questions!

T: He seemed to want to talk a lot. He was wringing his hands and his voice was very low at times and very negative and angry sounding at other times. He said a lot of negative things about the treatment.

B: I would too. I'm not convinced that chemotherapy is really any good. The patients get sick and die anyway. In fact, they are even sicker after they take the medicine than they are before.

D: I would die before I ever took it. No way. I'd rather die sooner, not by agonizing inches. Why prolong a life of agony?

M: I wouldn't want to live and cost my family lots of money. My husband and children have the rest of their lives to live. I don't want to be a burden on them. I have very strong feelings about what I want done. I want to be left to die as I choose.

G: You know, I don't feel the way you people feel. I think chemotherapy has some value, some good value. We just don't see the people who are living fairly normal lives out there while they're on therapy. I used to feel the way you feel, but I've talked with some patients who have had several good years, even though the medicine might not be working as well anymore when I see them.

M: Well, I suppose you're right. We only see the patients when they are hearing about their disease for the first time, or when they are sick again, often terminal or having to come back to the hospital for some special treatment like a blood transfusion.

B: But, look what it did to Mr. Leary. He was okay last week before he took that awful medicine Cis-platinum. Now, he has a fever of 103 and nothing seems to be helping him. I'm afraid he is not going to live much longer.

I feel terrible. He is such a nice person.

T: He is really great. But I don't believe it is the medication that has caused his temperature. That medicine doesn't do things like that. I wonder if he already had an infection, and it's just coincidence that it flared up at the time he received his first dose of the chemotherapy.

B: I never thought of that. Do you suppose that's possible?

G: I think so. They're doing all kinds of cultures to find out where his infection is located. The medicine couldn't cause the infection, but it might weaken his condition so it is harder for his system to handle it.

B: Maybe, but I still wouldn't have it for myself. Of course, others could take it if they wanted it. But not me, boy! Never!

Comments

In this exchange it is interesting to note that T and G had prior nursing experience (as L.P.N.s), while B, M and D had none. Often the student with more clinical experience is helpful to the less experienced student. It is also important to note that the students were expressing their feelings in a supportive atmosphere, using "I" messages and receiving acceptance without judgment. In addition, T described how she established and met her goal of being able to establish effective communication with her patient. She even received support and recognition for this from G.

EXERCISE 7: TEACHING THE PATIENT WITH CANCER OR ALTERED BODY IMAGE

Objectives—Cognitive

Students will

1. Review the principles of learning.
2. Discuss application of principles of learning to patient teaching.
3. Apply knowledge of therapeutic modalities employed with cancer patients or patients with altered body image.

Objectives—Affective

Students will

1. Share feelings regarding teaching needs of patients with cancer or altered body image.
2. Share feelings experienced while role playing patient or nurse-teacher.

Objectives—Psychomotor

Students will
1. Practice teaching skills.
2. Practice communication skills.
3. Practice role playing skills.

Confluent Techniques

Discussion group of ten students; diad; role playing; support groups of five students.

Description

1. (15 minutes) In discussion group of ten students, have students discuss objectives of exercise and review the major learning principles used in patient teaching:
   a. readiness
   b. motivation
   c. retention
   d. transfer
   Next, have them apply these principles to patient teaching by giving appropriate examples of each.
2. (5 minutes) Give directives for diad part of exercise. "Choose a partner preferably from your group. Each member of the diad will be given a different teaching situation. You are each to take five minutes to role play your teaching situation. Each student should take the role of the patient in one situation and the role of the nurse in the second situation."
3. (10 minutes) Teaching situations:
   a. Miss J, 22 years old, has Hodgkin's disease. She is about to start megavoltage radiotherapy. Your teaching is directed toward this treatment. What should she know about the effects of this therapy? What might her unasked questions be?
   b. Mrs. M, 45 years old, has just had a radical mastectomy. Your teaching goal is to help her adjust to her altered body image.
   c. Mr. L, 57 years old, has an above-the-knee amputation. He needs counseling regarding his altered body image and teaching about post-operative expectations and a prosthesis.
   d. Mrs. A, 23 years old, has acute lymphocytic leukemia. She is about to start on chemotherapy. Your teaching is directed at the effects of combination chemotherapy.
4. (15 minutes) Ask students to return to support groups of five students

to share their feelings regarding:

a. How the student role playing the patient felt about the teaching she received:
   (1) What was left out or unclear?
   (2) Was there a need for reinforcement in any area?
   (3) Did the nurse-teacher convey an empathic attitude?
   (4) Were learning principles observed?

b. How the student role playing the nurse felt about her teaching skills:
   (1) Was the teaching effective?
   (2) What might have made her teaching more effective?
   (3) Did she observe the principles of learning?
   (4) What affective response did she observe in the patient?

5. (10 minutes) Ask the students as a group to identify any obstacles to learning that may have been present during this exercise.

Sample Dialogue

Heather: When I was the lady with the mastectomy, I said I felt like a half a woman, and I was worried about my husband's reaction. Then Sara, as the nurse, told me, "Don't be silly; he didn't marry you for your body, he married you for you and you still are you." That made me mad.

Sara: Why? It's true isn't it?

Heather: Well, you as the nurse don't know that it is true. I felt like you didn't know what you were talking about.

Karen: Yes, you can't know. Maybe she had real cause to worry about her husband's reaction. Heather, what did you say to Sara?

Heather: Nothing really, I backed off and changed the subject.

Sara: Yes, she cut me right off. I was just trying to reassure her. I guess I jumped in with my own opinion and didn't really give her a chance to express her feelings.

Instructor: Can any of you think of a response that might have helped the patient express her feelings?

Susan: Well, suppose Sara used a reflective statement like, "You say you feel like half a woman."

Heather: Yes, then I might have had a chance to expand on that and tell you what I meant.

Sara: I guess I couldn't handle your feelings so I denied them and put you down for feeling that way.

Heather: Yes, I think that's what happened.

Instructor: Keeping this discussion in mind would you like to try to role play the situation again, trying a different approach on the nurse's part?

Sara and Heather: Yes.

Instructor: Okay. Perhaps the rest of the group could act as observers and offer constructive suggestions.

Comments

This was a well-developed group who handled role playing effectively. The members were open and honest with each other and were quite at ease sharing their feelings, using "I" messages. Their general attitude of trust and respect fostered much productive group activity. Sara was having problems with communication skills, both with her peers and her patients. Role playing offered the group an opportunity to observe her difficulties and provided a specific example on which the group could offer constructive feedback. The cohesiveness of the group afforded her the security she needed to respond objectively. The role playing experience provided a subtle, non-threatening means by which Sara was able to develop some beginning awareness of her communication problems.

EXERCISE 8: SEPTIC SHOCK INTERMIX

Objectives—Cognitive

Students will
1. Identify categories of patients who are at high risk for developing septic shock and the reasons.
2. Review pathophysiology of shock and physiological mechanisms of body compensation.
3. Describe pertinent signs and symptoms of septic shock, early versus late stages.
4. Explain rationale for methods used in resuscitating a patient suspected of going into septic shock.

Objectives—Affective

Students will
1. Share feelings related to responsibilities of the nurse in recognizing septic shock and providing prompt and vigorous intervention.
2. Be responsible for own individual and other group members' learning.

Objectives—Psychomotor

Students will
1. Practice attending skills.

2. Practice listening for content.
3. Practice paraphrasing.
4. Select a concept from assigned reading and teach it to another group member.

Confluent Techniques

Information intermix; diad; support groups of five students.

Class Preparation

Assign students to read the article: Taylor, C. When to anticipate septic shock. *Nursing 75* S(4): 34–38, 1975. Ask each student to select from this article a concept meaningful to herself, write it on a 3 x 5 card and bring it to class to share with other group members.

Post-clinical Conference

1. (1–2 minutes) Divide students into usual support groups.
2. (5 minutes) Allow time for sharing of concepts students brought with them. Notify groups when each minute or so is up, to assist them in allotting time for each member to share her concept.
3. (1–2 minutes) Have each student select a partner, not someone from her own group, decide who is A or B and sit facing each other.
4. (2 minutes) Assign A to teach B for one minute the concept that A brought on her 3 x 5 card. At end of one minute, students will switch roles and B will teach her concept to A.
5. (1–2 minutes) Ask students to switch diads, finding another partner who is not from her own support group.
6. (3–4 minutes) Direct students in this new diad to follow the same procedure as in Step 4, with some minor additions. This time, they will have 1½ minutes to teach their own concept, and in addition the one that they learned from their partner in the preceding diad. The brief time period encourages practice in condensing and paraphrasing information.
7. (5 minutes) Repeat Steps 5 and 6.
8. (1–2 minutes) Direct students to return to their original support groups.
9. (10 minutes) Ask each student to teach her group members the cumulative information she learned in her various diad situations.
10. (5 minutes) Have students compare and assess their original information with the total information they have gained.
11. (10 minutes) Ask students to share their feelings, new learnings, and reactions they had from this experience.

Comments

Information intermix as a format for conference discussion was described previously in the section on confluent techniques (see p. 115). We have used it with a variety of pertinent reading material. It has provided a valuable way for the students to practice counseling skills while learning cognitive content by teaching concepts.

EXERCISE 9: NEUROLOGICAL ASSESSMENT– CRANIAL NERVE TESTS

Objectives–Cognitive

Students will
1. Demonstrate knowledge of the normal function of the cranial nerves.
2. Discuss the pathological manifestations associated with dysfunction of the cranial nerves.

Objectives–Affective

Students will
1. Share feelings about the learning experience.
2. Develop group interdependence through pooling of knowledge.

Objectives–Psychomotor

Students will
1. Perform cranial nerve tests on other members of the group.
2. Demonstrate skillful use of ophthalmoscope, tongue blade, and so on, in testing the cranial nerves.

Confluent Techniques

Support groups of five students.

Class Preparation

All students are given a required reading assignment from the text on cranial nerve function and testing. Assign cranial nerve test exercise to students a few

days before it is to be done in post-clinical conference. Ask the students to assign the twelve cranial nerves among themselves and to come to the conference prepared to:
1. Discuss the normal function of the cranial nerve assigned to them.
2. Discuss the disease condition or pathology associated with nerve dysfunction.
3. Perform appropriate cranial nerve test(s) on the other group members.
4. Provide the necessary equipment for cranial nerve testing.
5. Answer any questions regarding assigned cranial nerve.

Post-clinical Conference: Cranial Nerve Testing Exercise

1. (2-3 minutes) Allow students time to assemble their testing equipment and divide into their support groups.
2. (30-40 minutes) Initiate student discussion of cranial nerve functions and demonstration and practice of cranial nerve tests.
3. (5-10 minutes) Ask total group of ten students to share their feelings regarding exercise.

Teacher's Guide

Observe students

1. Discuss the normal function of the nerve.
2. Discuss the disease condition(s) associated with dysfunction of the nerve.
3. Describe how the nerve is tested for functioning.
4. Demonstrate the test for nerve function on other members of the group.

Cranial Nerves
1st—Olfactory
  function: smell
  test: smell and identify various items, do each nostril separately
2nd—Optic
  function: visual acuity
  test: ophthalmoscope
3rd—Oculomotor
4th—Trochlear
5th—Trigeminal
  function: sensory fibers of face: ophthalmic, maxillary and mandibular branches
  tests: hot water, then cold water to chin
        pin test to various areas of face
        cotton wisp to cornea for response

6th—Abducens
   function of 3rd, 4th, and 6th: moves eyeball
   test for 3rd, 4th, and 6th: watch eye movements for symmetry using flashlight.
7th—Facial
   function: motor nerve of facial muscles
   tests: observe symmetry of facial movements
          identify taste of salt, sweet, sour, bitter
8th—Auditory
   function: vestibular, hearing, and balance
   tests: tuning fork (air and bone)
          balance: one foot and two feet
9th—Glossopharyngeal
   function: swallowing and taste on posterior one-third of tongue
   tests: taste on posterior one third of tongue
          tongue blade for gag reflex
10th—Vagus
   function: motor nerve of voluntary muscles of throat and larynx, decreases heart rate, supplies parasympathetic nerves to lungs, stomach, esophagus, and abdominal organs
   tests: tongue depressor
          check voice
          check symmetry of soft palate
11th—Spinal accessory
   function: motor nerve of sternomastoid and upper trapezius
   tests: turn and move head
          elevate shoulders
12th—Hypoglossal
   function: muscles of tongue
   test: check tongue movement

Comments

This is usually a very lively informative conference. The students especially enjoy performing the actual cranial nerve tests on each other, handling the ophthalmoscope, and being involved in an active learning situation. We have found that performance of the tests helps the students learn and remember the specific function of each cranial nerve. Since the presentation of the nerves is divided among the group members, the students are made more aware of their responsibility for the other members' learning and usually come to conference well prepared.

EXERCISE 10: SENSORY DEPRIVATION SIMULATION (LOSS OF SIGHT)

Objectives—Cognitive

Students will
1. Describe nursing intervention for patients with sensory deprivation.
2. Develop insight regarding the specific problems and needs of the blind person.

Objectives—Affective

Students will
1. Verbalize awareness of their own feelings when dealing with sensory deprivation.
2. Share feelings about dependency on another person.
3. Develop trusting relationship with peers.
4. Develop empathy for patients with sensory deprivation.

Objectives—Psychomotor

Students will
1. Simulate loss of sight.
2. Use all other senses to their fullest.
3. Demonstrate application of safety principles in order to provide security for a blind person.

Confluent Techniques

Diad; simulation; discussion group of ten students.

Description

1. (1–2 minutes) Ask students to select partners and form diads.
2. (5 minutes) Direct them to discuss with each other some personal experiences they have had in caring for patients with sensory deprivation.
3. (1–2 minutes) Give directions to students for their blindfolded trust walk.
4. (15 minutes) Direct Student A to lead Student B, who is blindfolded, around the building, up and down stairs, outdoors, and so on. Explain that students will: (1) select their own routes, (2) switch roles after five to seven minutes, and (3) return to class at the end of the second trust walk.

5. (5 minutes) Ask students in diads to share with their partners the feelings they experienced during the trust walk.
6. (5 minutes) Direct students to list effective ways to assist a person who is blind.
7. (1–2 minutes) Ask students to form one large circle.
8. (15 minutes) Request students to share their lists of ways to assist blind patients and to expand it to include patients with other sensory deprivations.
9. (10 minutes) Ask students to share their reactions and what they learned about themselves from this experience. They may use the following discussion guide if they so desire.
   Discussion Guide
   a. How did you feel about being blind?
      (1) Psychological response?
      (2) Behavioral response?
   b. What part of the experience was most anxiety-provoking? Least?
      (1) How did your anxiety manifest itself behaviorally?
      (2) What were the effects of your anxious behavior on your partner?
   c. How did you feel about your sighted partner?
   d. What actions on your partner's part were most helpful to you, the "blind" person?
   e. What did your other senses pick up?
      (1) hearing
      (2) tactile

Sample Dialogue

G: I felt really safe holding onto D. She led me around, and there was no problem, even with the stairs, until she led me from the cement sidewalk onto the grass. She didn't prepare me for this change. What a shock I felt go through me as my feet went from one texture to another. I felt undone. And you know, I do this same kind of thing all the time to my mother-in-law, who is blind. I could never understand her hesitancy when I was leading her around outdoors. Now I do. I understand better some of her fear. I won't lead her around without preparing her first for each change.

L: My hearing seemed much more important. I found myself listening harder. I was aware of all kinds of sounds that I probably don't usually pay attention to or even hear.

N: Going from shade to sunlight was really a significant difference for me. I noticed the difference in temperature, and I usually don't.

B: Some workmen near the outside door made some comments. I felt quite strange, helpless. I couldn't even see them. G had to tell me who they were. You know, describe them to me.

H: Well, I'm really upset. Someone touched me, suddenly without warning. She put her arm across in front of me, and I bumped into it. I jumped a mile and yelled at her, too. No one should ever do that to a person who can't see. It was obnoxious of that woman to frighten me that way. And she's a nurse, too. I don't think she should have interfered with what we were doing. She said something about trying to show me something, but I was too mad to listen to her.

W: Yes, I agree that can be very upsetting. I kept feeling that something was going to hit me in the face. I kept reaching a hand out in front of me to make sure that there was nothing there. Then I felt along the wall for security. It was awful when there was no wall, even though I had hold of L's hand. Imagine if someone had touched me when I wasn't expecting it. I would have been terrified.

D: I would rather be deaf than blind. I couldn't stand being in a total world of darkness with no end to it. At least we knew that this experience was going to end. Imagine if it wasn't going to.

L: But if you couldn't hear, you couldn't communicate very well. So much would be lost to live in a world of silence.

D: Yes, but even with being blind, your communication is hampered. You can't see people's expressions or what they are doing. And it would be so scary. You would lose your mobility.

W: To some extent, but look at Joe, the blind orderly. He gets all around the busy hospital faster than I do. And he doesn't bump into people either. He's an expert at using his cane. Maybe that takes the place of the wall that I needed to feel.

L: But never to hear voices, music, birds, sounds. . . .

M: True, but you can say that about blindness, too. Imagine having to count every stair to know when the end was coming, not to mention trying to find the edge of each step itself.

D: Well, lonely and isolated is how I felt.

M: Me, too, but also totally helpless and dependent.

G: It's scary to be in a world of darkness. Blindness. I'm not sure I would be able to cope with it.

Comments

The posture and physical behavior of the students, as they experience blindness, reflect their feelings of fear, insecurity, dependency, loss of control, anxiety, and isolation. Students experience excitement and enthusiasm as they gain insight into and empathy for problems and feelings of people who have sensory deprivations.

EXERCISE 11 : "NAME THAT DISEASE"

Objectives—Cognitive

Students will
1. Identify total symptomatic picture of a patient with specific disease process(es).
2. Determine laboratory data appropriate to disease process(es).
3. Assess nursing care needs of a patient presenting specific symptoms.
4. Formulate a nursing care plan to meet the patient's needs.

Objectives—Affective

Students will
1. Develop group cooperation and cohesiveness.
2. Share feeelings regarding the exercise.

Objectives—Psychomotor

Students will
1. Present a symptomatic case history to the other group of five students.
2. Listen to presentation of symptoms and, as a group, determine patient's diagnosis.

Confluent Techniques

Support group of five students; intergroup discussion.

Description

This exercise should be assigned toward the end of the semester so that the students are familiar with a wide variety of pathological conditions from which to choose. Each support group is instructed to choose a disease process, or two to three related disease processes. Each group must then prepare a patient case history including symptoms, laboratory data, pertinent social history, and so on, for a patient with this condition. All information, except the actual disease process, is assembled in logical order to be presented to the other support group, who must determine the patient's pathological condition. Then both groups formulate a nursing care plan to meet the patient's needs. When this is done, the second support group presents their patient history to the first group. Each group must choose a disease process that has been presented in class prior to the post-clinical conference.

Class Preparation

(5-15 minutes) A few days before assigned conference, explain the exercise directives and allow each group time to choose a disease process for their patient history and to divide the responsibilities for gathering appropriate data.

Post-Clinical Conference—Day of Exercise

1. (10-15 minutes) Instruct each support group to organize its patient history for presentation.
2. (10-15 minutes) Group 1 presents patient history to Group 2. Group 2 identifies disease and both groups formulate nursing care plan for the patient.
3. (10-15 minutes) Group 1 and Group 2 reverse roles and repeat Step 2.
4. (5 minutes) Both groups share feelings regarding the exercise, assess the completeness of the presentations, and evaluate intragroup cooperation.

Comments

The students usually work hard to present a complete symptomatic picture. They often include some irrelevant data to challenge the other group. They usually choose a combination of related pathological conditions to present. Intergroup competition is high during this exercise, as is intragroup cooperation. It is interesting to note the specific pertinent questions asked of the presenting group by the students who are trying to determine the disease process. This is an enjoyable exercise and an excellent way for students to assess and review the total symptomatic picture of a patient with a specific disease process and determine the appropriate nursing intervention.

EXERCISE 12 : I.V. THERAPY HANDS-ON EXPERIENCE

Objectives—Cognitive

Students will
1. Review signs of inflammation and infiltration of an I.V.
2. Use appropriate formulas to calculate proper drip rate.
3. Discuss nursing assessment of an I.V.
4. Review I.V. asepsis.
5. Review principles of I.V. therapy.
6. Discuss differences between various I.V. sets.
7. Review nursing action and principles employed when discontinuing an I.V.

Objectives—Affective

Students will
1. Share feelings regarding exercise.
2. Develop interdependence through pooling of knowledge.

Objectives—Psychomotor

Students will
Improve skills in adjusting, infusion rate, time-taping, and labeling I.V. bottles.

Confluent Techniques

Diads; simulation; group of ten students.

Description

Prior to clinical conference, the instructor sets up four stations, fully equipped with necessary I.V. apparatus, and a written directive of the learning task the student is to accomplish at each station.

Post-Clinical Conference

1. (2-3 minutes) Explain station set-up. Instruct students to work in diads and to follow directives at each station. Tell them they are to allow five to eight minutes at each station. Inform them the instructor will circulate and be available for answering questions or clarifying issues.
2. (40-45 minutes) I.V. hands-on exercise in diads.
3. (5 minutes) In large group of ten students, ask the members to share their feelings regarding the exercise.

Station Directives for I.V. Hands-on Conference

Station 1. Discuss areas to check and how to check them to assess if an I.V. is infusing without difficulty.

Site

1. Identify and describe signs of inflammation and infiltration.
2. What are the differences between inflammation and infiltration?
3. What action should you take when you discover one of these?

4. What is the problem with infiltration of some drugs into the tissue, e.g., nor-epinephrine (Levophed), KCl?
5. Write a SOAP note about this problem.

Type of solution.

1. Where do you check for the correct solution?
2. When do you check for the correct solution?
3. Discuss the differences between maintenance, replacement, and vehicle (KVO) I.V.s. Give examples you have seen in use.

Calculation problems.

1. 2500 cc of Normosol-M in 24 hrs: how many drops per minute?
2. 1000 Normosol-M and 500 Normosol-R in 24 hrs: how many drops per minute?
3. 350 cc Normosol-M in 24 hrs: how many drops per minute?
4. D5W KVO @ 100 cc/hr: how many drops per minute?
5. D5W in ¼ SS @ 125 cc/hr: how many drops per minute?

Station 2. Discuss areas to check and how to check them to assess if an I.V. is infusing without difficulty and on schedule.

Rate of infusion.

1. How do you figure out gtt per minute with an Abbott set for a microdrip chamber? For a macrodrip chamber?
   a. State the formula.
   b. State the number of gtt per cc for both micro and macro infusions.
2. State the steps involved in assessing whether an I.V. is ahead or behind or on schedule.
3. What is your responsibility for an I.V. that is ahead or behind or on schedule?
4. What is the maximum number of gtt per minute for an I.V. to infuse? For blood to infuse?
5. Practice time-taping a bottle.

Calculation problems.

1. You come on duty at 7:00 a.m. Mr. Smith's I.V. of 100 D5W was hung at 2:00 a.m. He is to receive 125 cc/hr. At 7:00 a.m. there are 500 cc left. The The I.V. is supposed to run for eight hours. How many gtt per minute will you adjust the I.V. to catch up?
2. Mrs. Brown's I.V. orders read: Isolyte H 1000 cc per 12 hours. It was started at 8:00 a.m. It is now 10:00 a.m. and 250 cc have been absorbed. What would your adjusted drip rate be?

Station 3.

1. Explain the application of each principle to the appropriate situation.

   Principles

   a. gravity
   b. displacement
   c. incompatibility
   d. osmosis
   e. diffusion
   f. size of tubing, size of vein, the larger the diameter of a tube the faster the rate of flow of fluid through it
   g. the higher the column of fluid the greater the pressure at the bottom

   Situation

   1. Pt. raising I.V. hand above his/her head: Could an air embolism occur?
   2. Pt. leaning on his/her hand with I.V. infusing.
   3. Pt. getting out of bed with an I.V. infusing.
   4. Raising or lowering I.V. bottle above the infusion site.
   5. Pt. with an I.V. infusing in the affected side.
   6. Tandem set-up (thru-and-thru). Which bottle empties first?
   7. Piggyback
   8. Pulmonary edema.
   9. Plugged air vent.
   10. Air embolism.

2. Set up a piggyback I.V. and discuss the principles involved.

   Calculation problems. The order reads Isolyte H 1000 cc per 8 hours.

1. How many gtt/minute?
2. The bottle is hung at 7:00 a.m. At 10:00 a.m., 500 cc has been absorbed. What would your drip rate adjustment be to make the bottle end on time at 3:00 p.m.?

Station 4. Discuss the method of discontinuing an I.V. How do you protect the vein? Why do you use a dry cotton ball and tape instead of alcohol wipe? How long is it necessary to apply pressure?

Piggyback

1. How do you regulate a piggyback?
2. Is it macro or micro?
3. How do you stop and record a piggyback?

Transfusion

1. What are the signs and symptoms of transfusion reaction? What is your responsibility when blood is first started?
2. How do you regulate blood?
3. Is it a macro- or microdrip?
4. How do you record blood?
5. What do you do when blood is discontinued or finished?

Infusion not running properly. What steps would you take when an infusion stops? (Try for ten or eleven steps.)

Asepsis. List areas of asepsis the nurse must maintain in I.V. therapy.

Hazards. What are the hazards of administering medications by an I.V. route? List three or four if you can.

Labeling. Check the label on the sample bottle. Does it have appropriate information?

REFERENCES

1. Egan, G. *You and Me: The Skills of Communicating and Relating to Others.* Monterey, Calif.: Brooks/Cole, 1977.
2. Ralston, S., and Hale, M. *Review and Application of Clinical Pharmacology.* Philadelphia, Lippincott, 1977.
3. Rogers, C. *Freedom to Learn.* Columbus, Ohio: Charles E. Merrill, 1969.
4. Stanford, G., and Roark, A. *Human Interaction in Education.* Boston: Allyn and Bacon, 1974.
5. Taylor, C. When to anticipate septic shock. *Nursing 75* 5(4):34 38, 1975.
6. Wooley, F.; Warnick, M.; Kane, R.; and Dyer, E. *Problem-oriented Nursing.* New York: Springer, 1974, pp. 110–115.

CHAPTER 7

And in Conclusion

Throughout this book we have attempted to acquaint the reader with the historical background of humanistic philosophy and its application to the educational process, specifically to nursing education. We have described the application of group process to a specific learning situation—the nursing clinical conference.

Perhaps our main goal in writing this book was not only to present a teaching method that has proved highly successful, but also to define and describe clearly the teacher's role in facilitating this method. The "how to" section in Chapter 6 will hopefully encourage the nurse educator to give group process a try.

We feel that, in concuding, we should present an evaluation of group process as a teaching and learning method. Therefore we have included in this chapter some student comments from evaluation questionnaires.

Before we present the students' comments, it might be of interest to the reader to know how we, as nurse educators, decided to use a humanistic group process approach in our teaching, as well as our personal evaluation of it. As our motivations and timing were different, we have decided to present our comments individually.

Virginia

I feel apprehensive and reluctant to share my personal feelings and evaluation of a confluent approach to teaching nursing students because everything that I can say is so overwhelmingly positive. It hardly seems that my evaluation could be that positive and be based on reality, yet it is.

Let me start by explaining that all my life I have experienced a didactic type of education, from elementary school through a graduate program in nursing. My feelings were never considered to be of value in the learning situation, only my intellect and my psychomotor performance of particular tasks. My feelings did not matter, as long as they did not interfere with my learning. I controlled them. I ignored them. In time, imitating my teachers, I, too, became a didactic teacher, a very didactic one. I was concerned about cognitive learning and mastery of appropriate subject matter. I was unaware of students' affective responses to learning.

One day during the time I was completing a postgraduate program in psychology and counseling, I met a woman, Dr. Marguerite Carroll, who was a different kind of teacher. She was not didactic. She did not use the old and familiar traditional approach that I knew so well. Instead, she facilitated the learning process. She did not lecture, yet, I was learning. And even better, I was excited and motivated to learn in a way I never had been before. Dr. Carroll used group process in such a way that all of us in her class were teachers and learners together. Confluence, the flowing together of mind and feelings, actually occurred. There was warmth, commitment, and a feeling of belonging that developed among the members of the class as we accepted responsibility for our own and each other's learning. I was excited by my own motivation and felt challenged to develop, grow, and learn as a whole person.

I wondered if I was the only one who felt so positively about Dr. Carroll's teaching. I talked with other students who were experiencing similar feelings. The consensus was that Dr. Carroll was a special teacher offering her students a special learning experience. I wanted more such learning experiences and eventually, I took every course that Dr. Carroll taught. I was never disappointed! My responses to learning under her confluent method in other courses were similar to those I had experienced in the first course. Always I learned as a whole person. The feelings that I experienced during learning were meaningful to me and important to share with my group members.

I began to want to use Dr. Carroll's approach in my own teaching. I was aware that some of the techniques that she used might work for me, but I needed more than techniques. I needed more awareness and understanding about Dr. Carroll's approach, but I was unsure of the specifics that I needed to learn. A solution for my problem appeared when Dr. Carroll offered a course entitled "Group Process in Education." I signed up for it immediately hoping to learn the secrets of her innovative approach to teaching.

Imagine my surprise when Dr. Carroll did not didactically reveal to any of us how to become facilitators of the learning process! Instead, we were responsible for developing and experimenting with our own plans for using group process in an educational setting of our own choosing. At the same time we were creating a confluent experience for students, we were learning how to do it in a confluent atmosphere facilitated by Dr. Carroll. She served as a role model, guide, resource person, group facilitator, and member of our group. It was in this group atmosphere that I experienced an understanding of what I needed to learn to become that kind of teacher; I am still learning more about this each day that I teach.

I did a lot of preparation and planning in getting ready to change my approach to teaching. I remember sharing with my classmates the misgivings and the sheer terror I had of not knowing what the outcome would be. What would happen when I let go of my didactic ways and implemented a confluent approach? Would it work? Would the students accept it? Would they accept me? Would they like learning this way? Would they learn as much? Was I different from them because I liked learning this way? Could I as a teacher, using group process, make confluence work for students or only enjoy it myself as a learner?

With the support of Dr. Carroll and my group members, I decided to take the risks and discover the outcome. It was the students' reactions to my initial attempt with a confluent appraoch that convinced me to continue in this direction. Their responses showed me that my move from being a didactic teacher to being a facilitator of the learning situation was a good one, for us all. They willingly shared their feelings about learning with this new approach:

—"I like this way. I learn a lot."
—"I feel relaxed."
—"I can ask questions of other students that I wouldn't ask you, and not feel embarrassed."
—"I get a chance to talk. I don't have to just listen."
—"I feel stimulated to learn."
—"I feel I'll remember more when I can read about it and then talk about it, too."
—"I feel you're not just checking up on me to see if I did my work, but that you're helping me to learn."
—"I feel closer to the other students now more than ever before. We stop and talk about situations, problems, experiences on the unit with other students that I wouldn't have before."
—"I feel that what I have to say is important."
—"If I've had a good day and am excited about learning, I can talk about it. Someone will listen. Also, if I've had a bad day, someone will listen. It's great for me."

My reaction to the student responses to my initial experiment with using a confluent approach was . . . euphoria! I had done it and not failed. I had been able to alter my approach to teaching and help students to have a positive experience with confluent education. I had not jeopardized their learning; I had enhanced it. Throughout the experiment, I had been terrified that students would think I was "copping out" by not directing and controlling the conferences with strong didactic leadership. I had always thought I was a good teacher, but this time I knew that I had guided and facilitated student learning better than I ever had before. I had reached them not only cognitively but also affectively. As I thought about this expereince, I became aware of the tremendous room for my own continous growth as a teacher and a person, which this approach had opened for me.

It became clear to me that previously in teaching nursing, I had only talked about treating patients as whole human beings, but now I was doing more than talking. In treating the students as whole human beings, through using confluence, I was providing them with a model for this behavior. In turn, I was becoming acutely aware of the students' awareness of their own feelings and those of their patients. Here are some of these feelings as I heard them expressed in group conferences and in individual conferences:

—"I feel really good. I did some teaching. I said this and the patient said . . ."
—"I talked with the patient. He had a tracheostomy and was barely understandable. It required extra time and patience to understand what he was trying to say. I taught him about his tube feeding. I wrote out speech exercises for him. I tried to understand and do what he wanted. He looked like he wanted to cry when I left. I felt like crying, too."
—"Do you ever get used to people dying? I felt so bad today. I felt hopeless and powerless to do anything to help my patient. I know he is dying." Another student responded, "I felt the same way when I came in to help you. Cancer has to be the worst disease possible. I feel so sad when I think about what it is doing to Mr. C." First student: "I don't know what to do with my feelings. Will I always feel this inadequate about being able to help when someone is dying? Will I get hardened? I don't really want that to happen. I want to show I care. I don't want to stop caring. But I don't want to be as torn as I feel right now."
—"I'm scared. An I.V. ran in too fast. The staff is concerned about the patient. I'm afraid something will happen to her. I watched the I.V. but not enough. I really messed things up. I feel awful."
—"When one of my patients became critically ill today, I had difficulty spending time talking with my other patient who also needed me. She needed someone to listen. I was frustrated and angry that there was not time or rather that I was unable to make time so I could sit and listen to her. She seemed upset about all the tests she is to have. She seemed scared and alone. I feel that I let her down."

As I listened to the students' affective responses to their learning experiences, I realized what I had been missing as a strictly didactic teacher. Since I had not been tuned into really listening to students, I had been unaware of their feelings and of their personal growth struggles. Using a confluent approach helped me become aware of these struggles and of the students' needs as whole individuals. I felt closer to each of them on a deeper level. I understood each of them better, and my teaching became more individualized. A new dimension was added to my teaching when I began to try to facilitate the affective growth as well as the cognitive growth of each student. Learning situations were no longer stagnant; they came alive. Students were interested and motivated, and I became a more interested and motivated teacher.

I feel as though I have come full circle, that a gestalt has been completed. I first experienced the importance of confluent education as a student. Later I read, studied, and talked about confluent education, trying to learn more about it. Eventually, I implemented a confluent approach in my own teaching. I have found that using this approach facilitates not only the growth of students, but my own personal growth as well. I have a feeling of satisfaction from completing this circle, and I feel good about this.

Since each student is different and each student group is different, however, there is a whole new challenge for continued growth and learning in each teaching/learning situation. I find accepting the challenge to be a little risky each time the process begins. I admit to feeling anxious each time at the beginning, wondering whether confluence will work again. It does. It is as electrifying with each group as it was with the first. I am more comfortable with using a confluent approach now. It is becoming a natural way for me to teach, and I appreciate the feeling of ease that time and expereince have brought. Would I ever exchange my confluent approach for my previous didactic one? Never. Confluence is good for me and it is good for students!

Norma

In attempting to relate my feelings, as a nursing instructor toward the use of group process as the teaching method employed in pre-clinical and post-clinical conference, I must first recall how I felt about clinical conferences before I start-using group process. Clinical conference, especially post-clinical, was frequently the low point of the clinical day for me and probably for my students as well. I would try to pull the day's clinical experience together by encouraging individual students to discuss their patients' diagnostic pathophysiology, nursing needs and so on. Then I would relate these presentations to the theoretical content focus for that week. The students sat waiting impatiently, ambivalently, or nervously (depending on their level of knowledge and self-confidence) to be called on. The better-informed, self-assured students talked on and one. The others usually offered a bare minumum of information. My role consisted of filling the gaps, asking pertinent leading questions and expanding on the information offered in order that approapriate content might be emphasized. I did most of the talking. The students expected me to do so and just sat back watching the clock, waiting for their "turn" to come and go. Very little sharing, listening, or learning took place. The students were bored, and I was extremely frustrated.

I finally decided my teaching methods must be changed if post-clinical conference was to become a meaningful learning experience. After some encouragement and guidance from a colleague, I decided to attempt a group process approach.

I must confess I undertook this endeavor with considerable trepidation. I need not have! While my first few conferences using group process were a bit uneven, as the students became more comfortable with the process and I stopped *teaching* and started *facilitating,* a most dramatic change took place. Post-clinical conference became an exciting, stimulating experience. The students thoroughly enjoyed being able to share meaningful clinical experiences in an informal voluntary way. They talked about issues that were relevant to themselves and to their learning needs. I began to see dynamic interactions in the small groups. They developed a positive group cohesiveness and began to demonstrate a genuine concern for each other's learning. They even began coming to post-clinical conference on time!

I think what I enjoy most about group process is the enthusiasm it generates. Each student becomes aware of her own worth and importance to the group, and this awareness fosters a desire to be an active participant. The drive to contribute to group learning motivates the student to prepare thoroughly for conference and willingly to share her research with the group. I see a supportive relationship among group members. If one is confused, the rest will pause and try to clarify. This type of behavior is supportive, caring—humanistic.

The group members become informed and involved with not only their own patients, but the patients for whom the other members are caring. They share clinical difficulties or successes they have experienced. They show a genuine interest in each group member's patients and often stop in on the clinical unit to say hello to the various patients for whom the group members are caring. The patients seem to enjoy this and have often commented on the friendliness and kindness the students have shown them, even the ones not directly responsible for their nursing care.

I have found the individual growth and awareness fostered by group process have affected my student-teacher rapport in a positive way. The students feel more secure about discussing problems, presenting their viewpoints, and sharing opinions with me. They no longer see me as the unapproachable, didactic teacher who stands before them and imparts "the word."

In all, I have found the use of group process rewarding, refreshing and stimulating. I look forward to post-clinical conference these days. I feel secure that the students are learning much more, with self-motivation and enthusiasm and from each other, then they ever learned from sitting and listening to me. My enthusiastic feelings for group process are further confirmed by direct student comments on clinical evaluation forms. The students' comments speak more strongly for group process as a teaching method than anything I could say.

As a teacher, I feel good about group process. I see it as a means by which students can grow intellectually and emotionally, develop self-awareness and confidence, improve their self-concept, and move toward the optimal goal of self-actualization. Furthermore, they can enjoy themselves and their classmates while learning and growing.

STUDENT EVALUATIONS OF GROUP PROCESS

The following are some actual comments that are typical of responses that students have made on the evaluative questionnaires. These comments are used by group members as a stimulus to discuss and evaluate how well they are working together and what areas may need some extra effort to improve their functioning as a group.

Questionnaire 1*

1. How effectively is the group working toward its goals?

   —"Pretty well—we usually get there when everyone really concentrates and sets their minds toward certain goals."
   —"We are compatible and work well together to attain goals."
   —"Sometimes we go off in other directions."
   —"We all seemed to gain different things from working together."
   —"Usually well prepared and works well together, giving time to all to speak and ask questions."

2. What problems does it seem to be having?

   —"Tend to get off on tangents and talk about things other than what we're supposed to be discussing."
   —"Sometimes we run out of time and not topic."
   —"Everyone gets a chance to talk, changing topics and moving on."
   —"Didn't learn too much at times. The group was kind of unprepared for discussions at times. It needed to be more organized."

3. Who is talking the most?

   —"All contribute equally."
   —"No one person. We take turns."
   —"Some days, one person talks more than others, but it seems to equal out, and we all do our fair share."

4. Who is talking the least?

   —"All speak equally."

5. What attempts are being made to include all members?

   —"If one person seems to be quiet, we ask her for her opinion or ask her to talk about her patient."
   —"Questions like 'what do you think?' are asked."
   —"We go around the group and everyone has a turn to talk. That way no one can monopolize."
   —"Has not been a problem. We all feel free to contribute at any time."

---

*Adapted from Stanford, G., and Roark, A. *Human Interaction in Education*. Boston: Allyn and Bacon, 1974. p. 121.

6. How does the group seem to feel about the task? About each other?

   —"Very compatible group."
   —"Everyone seems to respect each other and is willing to listen."
   —"I think everyone has taken a positive attitude to teach herself and each other."
   —"Mutual respect. It is a learning experience. If there is ill feeling, no one has shown any."

7. What might the group do to improve its effectiveness[1, p. 121]?

   —"The group should try to be more in-depth and more informative."
   —"Stop going off on tangents."
   —"Sit farther away from the other group—they are a distraction."
   —"I think it might be a good idea for groups to switch everyone once in a while or have the entire two groups meet together as one more often. The way it is now, the two groups become separate and segregated from each other."

Questionnaire 2*

1. Do you have a chance to talk as much as you want to?

   —"The group is very receptive to what I'm saying."
   —"The group members are congenial and courteous and allow all members to voice their opinions."
   —"Sometimes I think I tend to be too verbal and others don't get a chance to speak as much as they would probably like to."
   —"We have a dominating member, but I think if I asserted myself, maybe I could tone her down."
   —"Yes, except if time runs out, and the group has to break up."
   —"Usually, but I tend to think things through for a while before speaking, and then others are talking."
   —"Some people may dominate at times, but I'm sure I do, too."
   —"At times, when I have something to say, I can't because someone else is talking."
   —"Yes, one-to-one basis allows time for each person to participate (as we did today)."
   —"I feel I have to talk more than I want to; I must learn to wait out silence."

---

*Adapted from Stanford, G., and Roark, A. *Human Interaction in Education*. Boston: Allyn and Bacon, 1974. Pp. 121 124.

2. Are you happy during the discussions? If not, why not?

—"Yes, because there's a lot of new information learned from our discussion, and we have to correlate it more to our patients."
—"Yes, when the presentation is interesting and the conversation lively."
—"Yes, I enjoy the people in my group and feel at ease with them."
—"Yes, I pick up points that I missed during studying."
—"Yes, as long as I'm prepared and learn something new that interests me.'
—"Happy is an unusual word. I am comfortable in my group. We share common goals and interests."
—"Yes, because the group is able to work out the problems and come to a decision."
—"Most of the time. Sometimes I think that it is not that productive."
—"I enjoy teaching each other."
—"Except when we have discussions on interpersonal relationships. I find that difficult."
—"No, sometimes members go onto a different subject when we are supposed to be talking about one subject."

3. What could members of the group do to make you more satisfied during discussions?

—"More information and more in-depth discussion."
—"Relate more personal experiences about patient care."
—"I think we should try to stay on the subject."
—"Allow more equal talking time."
—"Include all members in the discussion."
—"Nothing, everyone participates in her own way."
—"Talk to the group and not the instructor."
—"Rely less on personal experience, or balance personal experience with classroom work."
—"At times, more enthusiasm and responsiveness."
—"Expand further when sharing knowledge."
—"Bring in new ideas from their experiences that would enlarge my knowledge of the subject."
—"Allow time to ask more questions to allow thorough comprehension of troublesome areas instead of re-teaching information already known."
—"I wouldn't alter them in any way."
—"I think they were fine."
—"My expectations were met more this half of the semester than at any other time in this program."

4. Does one person do most of the work of the group?

   —"We more or less contribute fairly to the discussion."
   —"Usually, two or three of the members are more knowledgeable and can offer more suggestions, but they do not monopolize the group."
   —"Not at all. We all seem to coax thoughts from each other."
   —"No, just some speak more than others."
   —"It depends who has had the most experience with the subject. In any group, someone always takes the position as the leader. Each person has her own role in the group in accordance to her personality."
   —"Everyone is prepared."
   —"Everyone in our group is very verbal."

5. When you speak, does everyone listen? If not, why not?

   —"Everyone listens and asks questions if they want to clarify a topic."
   —"Sometimes more than one person is talking at the same time, so you don't always listen."
   —"Yes, and I get feedback."
   —"Everyone is polite and listens to each other."
   —"Yes, unless there is a discrepancy."
   —"Usually, but many times I don't speak up or follow through on my point."
   —"I didn't get any clues that they weren't. If I did, I would try to be more presentable to the group as a whole."
   —"Everyone is able to express her views and is given equal time to do so."

6. Does everyone contribute toward the work of the group?

   —"Yes, although when one doesn't understand in complete depth the subject, one tends to ask lots of questions."
   —"Many times a member is shut out, very often by me. I would like to see this change."
   —"Some people have experienced more and so they can contribute more to the discussions."
   —"Everyone volunteers knowledge regarding the disease and patient care. If we have a question, we try to find the answer within our group."
   —"At times some students may be better prepared or have a better understanding of the material, but it seems to equal out."

7. What attempts are being made to include all members?

   —"Other members call on a person who has had a past experience with this kind of disease, and the others usually volunteer."
   —"Everyone has an opportunity to speak. No one monopolizes."

—"We question each other directly."
—"Members ask questions."
—"Most of the time by asking, 'What do you think?' 'Do we all agree?' 'It's your turn first this time.' "
—"Eye contact. Good listening skills."
—"We usually ask the opinions of everyone before we answer group questions."
—"We are beginning to ask each other what each one thinks."
—"We would say, 'Your turn to talk.' "
—"When someone has something to say, the others usually listen without interrupting. Usually each week a different person starts the talking."
—"If someone is quiet, we say, What do you think?' or 'Do you agree?' "

8. Does anything "bug" you during the discussions? If so, what?

—"I am sometimes overbearing and talk and overuse my time to talk."
—"Sometimes if I disagree with the correctness of the information, I find it frustrating."
"I would like to be able to ask more questions and have them answered either by the group or by a more knowledgeable person."
—"Two members of the group have more practical nursing experience than the other two. Occasionally, it appears they compete with each other in the amount of knowledge both have."
—"No, we had a good group and worked well together."
—"We need a bigger room for both groups."
—"Members who try to impress the instructor."
—"We do have a member who confuses issues. I don't know how to handle it. It doesn't bother me because I block it out, but it seems to bother other members."
—"Conflicts that are not resolved. Generally, I feel that group process is very effective and has helped me a great deal relating to people and working out problems as a team, which is important in nursing."

9. Is any one person most important to the work of the group?

—"No, everyone seems to work well together."
—"I think some are more vocal than others, but I do not think there is a leader."
—"The girls who are L.P.N.s can be very helpful by applying their experiences."
—"It depends on the information each person brings to the group (their patients, experiences for the day and so on)."
—"There is one who motivates us by her enthusiasm and mannerisms alone."

10. How effectively is the group working toward its goals?

    —"We are able to attain our goals."

    —"Everyone is coming prepared."

    —"We help each other to understand materials and provide positive reinforcement."

    —"Most of the subjects discussed are completed."

    —"If the goal is learning information, we are effective. If the goal is a group with members contributing fully, we need to work at it some more."

    —"Very effectively. The discussion often continues outside of class."

    —"If the goals are defined each time, each member works toward them. General discussion regarding patient care is a helpful learning tool if questions can be asked."

    —"I find our group discussing topics appropriate with our guidelines given by instructor. We are accomplishing what we set out to do, although sometimes we sidetrack, which is bound to happen!"

    —"Everyone is interested in the others' comprehension of material."

    —"We have mood swings. If the topic is an interesting new field, we respond and discuss."

    —"By and large, it's cohesive. Everyone shares freely and generously her information and knowledge. Most of the time, there is an attempt at reaching a consensus and a workable plan of action."

    —"We cover the clinical topics in-depth."

Terminal Questionnaire

We have found a terminal questionnaire, completed by the students at the end of the semester, to be a helpful tool. It affords us an opportunity to evaluate the success and limitations of the group process experience. It also allows the student an opportunity to review and assess her semester's learning experience.

The following is the terminal questionnaire we use, with students' comments included.

1. Do you like group process as a form of post-clinical conference?

    —"Definitely. I feel comfortable enough to say what I am feeling, and, because I can ventilate and realize that other people are experiencing what I am feeling, I feel less anxious."

    —"Yes, it's been the most constructive post-clinical conference experience I've had so far."

    —"Definitely. I learn from the factual information contributed by members. I also gain insight into personalities and member interactions. Analyzing roles is enlightening (and fun). It is interesting to see the changes that occur in group interactions when a member is not present because of rotating, etc. I learned a lot about people in general."

—"For the first time I am learning something at post-clinical conference. I have also become more aware of others in respect to their ideas, levels of intelligence, cognitive processes, and personalities. I also like group process because all participate and ask questions. I don't feel alone."

—"At first I didn't like being 'pushed' into it. But we were able to ventilate our feelings, which helped. I feel very satisfied with my personal growth (I gained a lot of insight about myself through group process). And I feel I was able to gain knowledge and apply it clinically. I'm beginning to feel like a nurse. I feel I learned a lot about patient teaching. I know this was my weak point at the beginning of the semester."

—"I like group process in general."

—"I like to hear other students interpretations of readings and problems and how they handled a situation."

—"At first I didn't, but I have found that it has made me more aware of my feelings and thoughts, not just with patients but with other people that I converse with."

—"It's teaching me to be more self-assertive in a 'civilized' way."

—"It lets you discuss problems in a small group and get the reactions of other members."

—"I think it's important in our learning to communicate effectively with others."

—"I feel it has helped me in learning and interacting with people."

—"At times I feel the group gets stale. Perhaps we could have a few more dynamic group sessions with outside speakers or demonstration sessions with various personnel."

—"Yes and no. I feel that it is not the most effective means of learning. It is all right occasionally, but consistently, I find it boring."

—"This allows both students and clinical instructor to explore new knowledge and learn about things together."

—"It gives everyone a chance to participate instead of just listening to one person or instructor. It gets you more involved, and by doing so you learn more because you retain it better."

—"I find that talking to the group in post-clinical conference helps us to learn more from each other."

—"I enjoy hearing other people's experiences; sometimes they express feelings that I too am feeling."

—"Everyone feels more at ease and under less pressure of the instructor zeroing in on one person, as opposed to everyone in a group."

—"This is a new experience that I am enjoying, although I do feel that we need more guidance in some areas (through lectures) concerning EKGs, acid base balance, and so on. I would like also to discuss more articles that deal with difficult subjects so that we may go through them with each other and reinforce the learned (or confused) subject."

—"The time that is given in both pre-clinical and post-clinical conferences was well spent in learning compared to my previous experiences in the program, where a lot of times were a waste of time."

2. What problems did the group have in functioning?

—"By and large, we work well together. This seems to be related to the degree of fatigue experienced by each member, all of whom are very verbal. Tempers seem to be short at the end of the day, but we seem to be able to apologize for behavior and go on."

—"When all are tired, we aren't very productive."

—"I don't think we're as organized as we could be. We seem to get off the track."

—"Sometimes, there are conflicts and the group can't make one decision."

—"Some lack of enthusiasm. I think such a small group, week after week, has periods of becoming stale."

—"We need more time to express ourselves fully."

—"It can be confusing when different people disagree on answers or information."

—"Discussion falls off before it reaches depth."

—"Sometimes, our pre-clinical conferences are repetitious, e.g., orthopedics!"

—"Distraction by the other group."

—"You get out of it what you put into it."

—"Maybe coping with our 'problem member,' but we are managing better there."

—"Lack of questioning each other."

—"Getting started."

—"Occasional personal conflicts."

3. What could the group have done to improve its functioning?

—"Give more in-depth information."

—"Stick to the subject."

—"The instructor should join us once in a while as leader."

—"Have a larger room so we could sit farther away from the other group."

—"Set a specific time to end so that everyone knows the amount of time they may have to speak."

—"Take time to learn to cope with our 'problem member.' "

—"Try to be open and honest with each other."

—"Make more of an effort to include all members."

—"Ask each other questions regarding whatever is not understood."

—"Not to hesitate sharing personal learning experience. I feel sometimes

we don't want people to think we didn't know, so we remain silent."
—"Keep goal in mind, firmly. Mix book learning with practical experience better. Perhaps read up more on background information when needed."
—"Make sure everything that's supposed to be covered in discussion is covered."
—"Weigh out both sides."
—"Divide work up among members and combine it at conferences, allowing for discussions and new views on solving problems."
—"On occasion, everyone tends to get upset if someone doesn't agree. I feel if the person can assess what she believes and also what the other member of the group believes, this would increase the successful functioning of group process."

4. What did you enjoy the most about group process?

—"The sharing that occurred among us—feeling of support developed."
—"Self-teaching and peer teaching."
—"It is so nice to learn by discussing material with other students instead of being lectured to. It was the first clinical experience that I learned so so much in and enjoyed so much. I learned how to communicate with a group of people."
—"I like the closeness that resulted. I also liked the freedom to exchange information without feeling that one was trying to upstage the other."
—"Sharing information with peers is for me the most advantageous way of learning. We knew also that we had to teach, so we did our best to get all the information we needed. We became very cohesive and worked well together."
—"Five heads are better than one. Through group process, by listening to others' thoughts and ideas, I learned far more than I would have on my own and also heard different ideas on how to approach a problem."
—"Pooling information and ideas toward a better understanding. Role playing was very helpful."
—"Learned very much from it and felt it a better learning experience than teacher-to-student."
—"It allows everyone to participate. It allows for a better thought process because you can state ideas, talk them over and restate them."
—"No one person was singled out. Everyone had opportunities to speak and everyone felt very comfortable."
—"It helped me, in that I was able to share with other members of the group any problems I was having."

—"Learning to communicate with others. Talking things over helps one to absorb information better."
—"At first I hated group process. I couldn't accept that we could all have

our own opinions. I thought we were all supposed to have the same answers. But I learned to work with others better."

—"Like the exchange of information that takes place, another means of learning and adding to store of knowledge. One learns the difference between withdrawal and aggression."

—"Being able to talk about my anxiety and knowing that others had the same problem."

—"That we were able to get to know each other better and since everything comes from a different view, everyone was able to contribute to the learning process."

—"I looked forward to group and post-clinical conference where I had not before. I found I had actually learned something and wasn't watching my watch to see how much longer I had to go until I could leave."

—"First of all, since we were in small groups and were able to talk together, questions could be asked without feeling embarassed. Therefore, more questions were asked and more situations were made clear. Since we taught each other in some instances, what we learned stayed in our minds and wasn't forgotten, compared to a teacher giving us information that we would write down and probably forget. When we did the research and then taught each other or discussed it with each other, we were reinforcing it in our own minds. It also gave us a feeling of independence and self-worth."

—"I also enjoyed group for the reason that everyone got to know one another and to feel closer. Previous to group, no one got to really talk to each other and get to know each other. It also gave the students a chance to be heard, to talk about a problem they were having and to realize that someone else may have been going through the same thing. Group also made me feel more relaxed and confident on the floor and improved my nursing care, since we had discussed some of it in conference, and I was better able to understand my patient's diagnosis, symptoms, and medical treatments."

—"Other activities such as one-to-one teaching were also useful as the student had to have listening skills and have her thought processes at work. In a normal conference with the instructor leading the discussion, there is a tendency on the part of the student, particularly if she's tired after being on the floor, to daydream and not pay attention. You don't do that with group process—it would be too obvious! Plus, you're more stimulated when you know you're going to participate."

—"Once I was on a more intimate level with my fellow classmates that were in my group, I felt very comfortable and was able to express my thoughts and feelings. Also, if I didn't understand something, e.g., a certain medication, I didn't feel embarrassed to ask to go over it one more time. I learned a lot from my fellow classmates, and it also gave me a chance to show my knowledge, knowledge I wasn't aware I had retained, giving me confidence. I feel very positive toward group process as a beneficial learning experience. It really made me prepare for assignments and get down to work, rather than sleep through a lecture."

"AND IN CONCLUSION"

Earlier chapters have explained our belief that humanizing nursing education is a step that must be accomplished in order to produce humanistic, self-actualizing nurses who will be able to accomplish satisfactory changes in nursing practice and provide humanistic health care to people. Using a confluent approach to nursing education through the method of group process has allowed us to begin to take up this challenge

We find group process to be an excellent vehicle for enabling us to implement confluence and enhance effective and dynamic communication between ourselves and students and among students themselves. It enables us to apply principles developed by humanistic psychology that assist the process of a person's adaptation to the world around her or him. Group process brings together the affective, cognitive, and psychomotor realms of learning into a total dynamic experience. This type of experience humanizes nursing education by promoting the development of the whole student toward self-actualization. It exerts a positive influence on the development of the teacher as well. The results are intellectual and personal growth for everyone concerned.

For us as nurse educators, applying a learning theory that combines the principles of Gestalt therapy, concepts of confluent education, and group process has been fascinating, at times frustrating, but nonetheless a rewarding and satisfying experience. We are excited by our belief that this approach holds enormous potential for eventually humanizing the health care delivery system. This is possible, however, only if everybody is willing to join in this effort. If this happens, then the dream of humanizing nursing education can become a reality! We hope that this book has provided some of the background necessary to enable the reader to join with us in further developing, refining, and applying this approach in nursing education.

We as educators will need to document, through systematic research, the effect that this humanizing process has on the learning experiences of nursing students and teachers. Once this work is completed, we will need to assess the long-range effects that it has on humanizing nursing practice and the health care system. Hopefully, with your help, energy, and effort, our ultimate goal of contributing toward humanizing the delivery of health services to people will be realized.

REFERENCE

1. Stanford, G., and Roark, A. *Human Interaction in Education.* Boston: Allyn and Bacon, 1974.

Index